T0146202

Living in Death's Shadow

Living in Death's Shadow

Family Experiences of Terminal Care

and Irreplaceable Loss

Emily K. Abel

JOHNS HOPKINS UNIVERSITY PRESS   BALTIMORE

© 2017 Johns Hopkins University Press
All rights reserved. Published 2017
Printed in the United States of America on acid-free paper
9 8 7 6 5 4 3 2 1

Johns Hopkins University Press
2715 North Charles Street
Baltimore, Maryland 21218-4363
www.press.jhu.edu

Library of Congress Cataloging-in-Publication Data

Names: Abel, Emily K., author.
Title: Living in death's shadow : family experiences of terminal care and
    irreplaceable loss / Emily K. Abel.
Description: Baltimore : Johns Hopkins University Press, 2017. | Includes
    bibliographical references and index.
Identifiers: LCCN 2016019645 | ISBN 9781421421841 (hardcover : alk. paper) |
    ISBN 1421421844 (hardcover : alk. paper) | ISBN 9781421421858 (electronic) |
    ISBN 1421421852 (electronic)
Subjects: | MESH: Terminal Care | Grief | Attitude to Death | Family Relations |
    Chronic Disease—psychology | Caregivers—psychology | United States |
    Personal Narratives
Classification: LCC R726.8 | NLM WB 310 | DDC 616.02/9—dc23
    LC record available at https://lccn.loc.gov/2016019645

A catalog record for this book is available from the British Library.

*Special discounts are available for bulk purchases of this book. For more information,
please contact Special Sales at 410-516-6936 or specialsales@press.jhu.edu.*

Johns Hopkins University Press uses environmentally friendly book materials,
including recycled text paper that is composed of at least 30 percent post-consumer
waste, whenever possible.

Contents

Living in Death's Shadow

Introduction

"Living for a long time with fatal illness is still a new cultural phenomenon," writes physician Joanne Lynn, "and we have much to learn about how to make this time of life comfortable and rewarding for patients and families." Because degenerative, chronic conditions have replaced acute diseases as the major cause of mortality, large numbers of people live in death's shadow for months or years. "My father started dying twenty years before he actually died," recalled one adult daughter. After his heart attack and bypass surgery, the specter of his death "floated above us at all times." Such an experience has no place in the many recent movies, television series, magazine articles, and books that have helped to heighten popular awareness of the end of life. Debates about "do not resuscitate" orders, euthanasia, and the termination of life-prolonging technologies dominate the media, leaving little room for conversations about the equally contentious and consequential issues that arise throughout the long course of dying.[1]

Memoirs by kin (including families of choice as well as those of origin) help to fill the knowledge gap. This book relies on 105 narratives by family members of people who died from chronic disease after 1965. The chapters examine the common experience of people confronting serious chronic disease, including learning the diagnosis, grappling with the decision whether to enroll in a clinical trial, acknowledging the limits of medicine, receiving care at home and in health care institutions, and, finally, obtaining palliative care. The book challenges three of the common assumptions that surround stories of death and dying in the modern age. One is that patient autonomy has steadily increased and that its expansion always represents progress. Developments contributing to that belief include the demand that physicians tell the truth about diagnoses and prognoses, the passage of regulations mandating that physicians obtain permission from patients for medical procedures, and the rapid expansion of both popular medical information and advance directives. But some patients and family members try to shut out the bad news that doctors deliver, many physicians continue to conceal hopeless diagnoses, and popular health websites, articles, and manuals do not necessarily diminish physician status and authority.[2]

The overriding emphasis on individual autonomy presents other difficulties as well. The concept is closely associated with personal control; thus, proponents of encouraging advance directives and legalizing physician-assisted suicide often present them as ways to enhance individual choice. But many family members of dying people gradually become aware of the fragility of life and the randomness of fate. The "ethic of care" formulated by feminist philosophers challenges the focus on autonomy in another way. As Virginia Held writes, that ethic views "persons as interdependent rather than as independent individuals and holds that morality should address issues of caring and empathy and relationships between people rather than only or primarily the rational decisions of solitary moral agents." Memoirs depicting the intimate connections between patients and their families underline that point.[3]

The memoirs also question the exalted value increasingly assigned to the acceptance of mortality. Critics of aggressive, high-intensity services at the end of life often stress the importance of acceptance. They note that people who acknowledge the inevitability of death are less likely to insist on expensive and ultimately futile treatments. In addition, an understanding of the finite nature of human existence can help to endow all of life with greater meaning. But acceptance often becomes the new imperative, demanding that both dying individuals and the people closest to them mold their emotional responses to conform to a precise script.

Finally, the book cautions us against trying to shift the site of death during a period of hostility to government services. A central concern of the movement to humanize death is to enable more people to die at home. As advocates argue, most people want to be at home at the time of death, but relatively few actually are; many patients who spend their last days in intensive care units (ICUs) receive unwanted and unnecessary treatment; and changes in the reimbursement structures of both Medicare and Medicaid would allow those programs to provide far more home-based care. But care for people at the very end of life tends to be especially difficult. Obituaries frequently report that an individual died peacefully at home surrounded by loved ones. The reality, however, may have been quite different. Dying people often experience nausea, breathlessness, and excruciating pain (which medication cannot control), become paranoid and delusional, and display physical symptoms that can be viewed as repulsive. Many families are ill equipped to deal with these troubles without enormous amounts of support.

In addition to unsettling these three widespread assumptions, this book exposes the lack of attention to the myriad difficulties encountered throughout the long course of a serious chronic disease. I began this project expecting the memoirs to provide a wealth of information about initiating cardiac resuscitation attempts and withholding or withdrawing life support technologies. Those issues dominate public discourse about death and dying. Acting as surrogates for incompetent patients, many family members are the ones who must make the most critical decisions. Studies suggest that, especially when patients have not made their wishes clear, those relatives often experience high levels of confusion and guilt after the patient's death. Just two of the memoirs I collected, however, discussed struggling to decide whether to "let" someone "go." Four writers noted that patients had tried to end their own lives, but only one discussed family responses to that decision. Another few mentioned signing "do not resuscitate" orders at a doctor's behest or because doing so was a precondition of enrolling a relative in a nursing home. In the great majority of cases, questions about treatment at the very end of life appeared relatively minor when considered within the entire sweep of a long-term fatal disease. As a result, I focus on issues that seemed more important.[4]

The book begins in the mid-1960s, when a series of developments began to transform the experiences of dying people and those closest to them. The first was the 1965 passage of Medicare and Medicaid. By placing much of the cost of the care of people with terminal illnesses on the government, those programs made decisions about how to die more political and public. The programs also helped to shift the site of death, first from homes to medical institutions and then back to the home. Today, when Medicare covers more than 80 percent of people who die and Medicaid is the major payer for long-term care, numerous commentators argue that the financial incentives of both programs distort the care provided to people in the last phase of life.[5]

Two additional developments affected mortality in contradictory ways. One was the growing dominance of ICUs and associated technologies.

Although ICUs began as rooms where special nurses congregated, they increasingly became the site for high-tech interventions. By the mid-1960s, defibrillators, feeding tubes, and respirators filled the units. As new technologies have continued to emerge, a growing proportion of patients have received high-tech medical services near the end of life.[6]

The other was the rise of a movement to humanize the care of dying people. By the late 1950s, a growing number of academics and health professionals began to criticize medicine's overriding emphasis on recovery and cure, the secrecy surrounding dire diagnoses and prognoses, and the lack of attention to the needs of patients approaching finality. The 1969 publication of Elisabeth Kübler-Ross's *On Death and Dying* helped to spread those ideas to a broad public. Her most famous and controversial contribution was her theory of the stages of grief, through which, she argued, both patients and family members passed. The book quickly became an international best seller, with more than a million copies purchased by 1976, and it has never been out of print.[7]

My book contributes to a growing literature on the patients' perspective. Three landmark works helped to shape that field. In sociolinguist Elliot G. Mishler's 1984 book *The Discourse of Medicine: Dialectics of Medical Interviews*, he analyzed communication between doctors and patients, showing how the voice of the doctor continually drowns out that of the patient. The following year historian Roy Porter enjoined his colleagues to "lower" their "gaze" from doctors and hospitals "onto the sufferers." And 1988 saw the appearance of *The Illness Narratives: Suffering, Healing, and the Human Condition*, by psychiatrist and anthropologist Arthur Kleinman, urging physicians to listen to patients' stories to understand better how they make sense of their troubles. Since that time, there has been a flowering of personal narratives of illness and disability as well as works by health professionals and scholars in various fields seeking to illuminate the patient's point of view. The narratives used in my study, in contrast, examine patients through the eyes of their family members.[8]

Although most people are embedded in social networks, the attention directed toward patients has not extended to their families. A rapidly proliferating literature addresses the services family members render as caregivers, but other aspects of their experience receive short shrift. Relatives typically share dying people's hopes, fears, and disappointments. They, too, must make decisions under conditions of uncertainty and confront the approach of death. And most simultaneously sustain intimates and witness their deterioration.[9]

Like the health care system, families underwent a major transformation beginning in the mid-1960s. As both longevity and childlessness increased, families came to include a higher proportion of elderly people. The number of housewives dramatically declined as more and more women entered the labor force. Families also became less uniform and stable. The rate of both divorces and remarriages rose, and a growing number of people cohabitated outside marriage. New family forms recently have emerged as a result of the legalization of gay marriage and the growing use of reproductive technologies, especially surrogacy and donor insemination.[10]

Health policies directed toward families historically have relied less on statistics about their shape and structure than on the assumptions of medical providers. Throughout the nineteenth century, professional rewards and privileges eluded doctors. Without the ability to regulate access, "regular" doctors could not easily distinguish themselves from unorthodox practitioners. Moreover, the great majority of physicians worked in homes, where they were exposed to lay scrutiny. Career success depended on the judgment not of peers but of family members and friends. Although doctors at the beginning of their careers were especially likely to feel intimidated, even experienced doctors could not claim superior competence. Doctors and family caregivers (most of the latter women) employed many of the same diagnostic and therapeutic practices. In addition, nineteenth-century medical beliefs encouraged doctors to value personal ties both to alleviate stress and as a source of medical knowledge.[11]

Insecure about the value of their training, especially vis-à-vis women who assumed the right to judge medical skills and to direct treatment, physicians responded in various ways. Many routinely disparaged women's knowledge and skills, complaining about ignorant ladies. One doctor condemned "the old grannies who thought they knew more than the physician. To us doctors on the frontier these ancient know-it-alls were often a positive curse." Doctors also portrayed the bedside gathering of friends and family as a threat to the patient rather than a source of comfort and support. Arguing that family and friends disturbed and alarmed patients, doctors sought to exclude sickroom visitors. Others gradually shifted their practices to offices.[12]

At the turn of the twentieth century, doctors succeeded in usurping women's authority at the bedside. Aligning themselves with dramatic medical advances, "regular" physicians were able to assert dominance over other practitioners as well as family caregivers. They also could more easily denigrate family caregivers. Discovery of the bacteriologic causes of specific diseases made it more acceptable for physicians to maintain distance from patients. The shift to hospitals as the site of medical training reinforced emotional distance. "In the hospital," historian Kenneth M. Ludmerer wrote, patients were "detached from their home, place of work, friends, and family." Medical schools emphasized the importance of maintaining emotional distance from patients, not developing intimate ties with them. Although nurses never were considered the equals of doctors, they, too, sought professional status by donning the mantle of science and cultivating emotional detachment. As the number of nursing schools rose, nursing leaders defined their occupation in terms of technical skills and abstract knowledge.[13]

By the late twentieth century, growing concerns about the impersonality and cost of health care encouraged new respect for family members. Returning care to the home increasingly was justified on both humanitarian and economic grounds. Nevertheless, many attitudes from the nineteenth century remain widespread today. In the world of health care delivery, Carol Levine and Connie Zuckerman wrote, "families are at best tolerated or sometimes accommodated, at worst patronized or labeled as barriers to good patient care. Hospital administrators consider families, like labor relations and risk avoidance, difficult 'management' problems." Clinicians continue to deprecate the personalized knowledge of family members while claiming to monopolize technical and medical expertise. Contending that families are more likely to be suffused with rancor than warmth and solicitude, doctors argue that they are best equipped to make decisions about patient welfare. And the growing visibility of malpractice suits has intensified fears of lay scrutiny.[14]

In contrast to illness narratives by patients, those by family members have received little scrutiny. Some of the memoirs used in this study appeared as journal articles or book chapters. In a few cases, the discussion of a relative's illness and death represented a small section of a book devoted to another topic. In many more cases, the memoirs were published as full-length books, describing the experiences of both patients and family members in lavish detail.[15]

The most common diseases discussed were cancer (53 memoirs), Alzheimer's disease and related dementias (30), and AIDS (16). Smaller numbers of memoirs described people with cystic fibrosis, multiple sclerosis, amyotrophic lateral sclerosis (ALS), heart disease, and emphysema. Eighty-seven of the patients were adults at the time of diagnosis; the other eighteen were children. Because women tend to be more involved than men in caring for sick and dying relatives, it is not surprising that 72 percent of the writers were women. That figure included 34 daughters, 20 mothers, 17 wives, 1 sister, 1 female partner, 1 daughter-in-law, 1 niece, and 1 woman who considered herself extended kin. The male authors included 13 sons, 7 husbands, 4 fathers, 4 male partners, and 1 brother.

Like other memoir writers, the authors of these narratives were overwhelmingly white, well educated, and relatively prosperous. A high proportion were writers, journalists, and academics. Some were extremely prominent. As social inequality grows, the experiences of members of different groups increasingly diverge. Members of privileged populations tend to be less religious than others, less likely to defer to medical authority, and more likely to consider themselves qualified to seek medical information on their own. We can assume, therefore, that many of my generalizations apply only to people with high social status. Of course, even people with good incomes and substantial resources often have difficulty paying for health care. The author of one memoir, a woman whose son died after a thirteen-month struggle with a brain tumor, wrote that after his funeral she and her husband had exhausted their resources. In many other cases, financial considerations dictated health care decisions. The great majority of writers, however, had access to what they considered good care.[16]

Most memoirs included here were recently published: 10 appeared between 1970 and 1979, 15 between 1980 and 1989, 27 between 1990 and 1999, 26 between 2000 and 2009, and 27 between 2010 and 2014. The publication dates reflect the rapid proliferation of memoirs since the 1970s. Between 2004 and 2005, the sales of memoirs grew more than 400 percent. In 2010, Daniel Mendelsohn, himself the author of a well-known memoir, referred to "this confessional age, in which memoirs and personal revelations tumble out in unprecedented abundance."[17]

As memoirs flood the market, they come under increasing attack. A rash of articles, mostly by literary critics, charge that too many memoirs are published, that the authors include ordinary people as well as accomplished writers and celebrated individuals, and that, rather than presenting unmediated truth, they provide only one point of view. In a widely cited diatribe in the *New York Times Book Review,* Neil Genzlinger wrote that the list of authors who previously would be considered "memoir-eligible" is "lost in a sea of people you've never heard of, writing uninterestingly about the unexceptional, apparently not realizing how commonplace their little wrinkle is or how many other people have already written about it. Memoirs have been disgorged by virtually everyone who has ever had cancer, been anorexic, battled depression, lost weight."[18]

But what literary critics view as problems, many historians and other social scientists may regard as gifts. The large number of published memoirs grants us easy access to a broad array of sources. Even when we do not seek representative samples, we tend to be especially interested in the "unexceptional." And memoirs are valuable to us precisely because they offer the perspective of particular individuals. "Disassembling objectively known events and facts," historian Paula Fass writes, "the memoir reminds us that people remain the fundamental unit of historical experience and they are sentient beings, not simply masses of faceless humanity." In this book I often quote from conversations the authors have reconstituted or refer to events they claim to have experienced, but my major goal is to discover how the memoirists understood those events.[19]

Literary critics challenge the motivations of memoir writers as well as their products. A common assertion is that the authors confuse public confession with private therapy, want to view themselves as victims, and are unforgivably self-absorbed. Although some authors of the memoirs included in this study may have fit that description, most wrote for other reasons as well. One was to try to heal a rupture. Sociologist Arthur W. Frank writes that people need "new stories" when "disease disrupts the old stories." Edward Hirsch, a poet and the president of the John Simon Guggenheim Foundation, referred to the night before he learned of his son's death as "the last night of my old life." A mother dramatized the moment she learned that her adolescent son had leukemia: "A tremendous bolt split the world." Other memoir writers described themselves as being in a new land. Anne Sexton famously wrote, "In another country, people die." The father of a young man with metastatic cancer noted that when his son's wife heard the fatal diagnosis, "she crossed from one country into another." Writing memoirs helped some authors make sense of the family catastrophe, connecting past and present in a meaningful way.[20]

In addition, many writers wanted to pay tribute to or "memorialize" the relative who had died. That motivation seemed especially intense in three situations. Parents who had experienced the death of a child wanted to demonstrate that their child's life had had meaning despite its premature end. Spouses and children of people with dementia wanted to recall the person they felt they had lost over many years. And mothers of young men who had died of AIDS wanted to show that their sons were uniquely precious human beings despite the stigma surrounding the disease. Closely related was the desire to write counternarratives, challenging the portrayal of very sick and dying people in medical discourse. Many authors complained that health professionals had reduced patients to data gleaned from CAT scans, MRIs, X-rays, and biopsies. The writers sought to reclaim their memories of loved ones, telling stories about whole people, with distinctive characteristics, histories, and life circumstances.[21]

Some writers also wanted to share what they had learned. As the author of a recent book on post-traumatic stress disorder notes, "Trauma, which obviously leads to great pain, can also lead to deeper knowledge about human existence." Having lived most of their lives denying their transience, the memoirists suddenly understood that serious illness can strike anyone at any time and that death eventually comes to us all. Stephen S. Rosenfeld, whose parents had died of cancer within six months of each other, wrote that the experience forced him to think "about the possibilities of human existence in categories that previously had been strange to me. This is what ultimately defined the time of their dying." His memoir about their deaths enabled him to disseminate his new awareness. Perhaps because the death of a child is the most terrible tragedy most of us can imagine, parents who had experienced that loss were most likely to claim special knowledge. Emily Rapp wrote a wrenching account about caring for a baby with a fatal degenerative disorder. After describing conversations with the other parents of terminally ill children, Rapp commented, "The experience of being Ronan's mom was not, I grew to learn, without wisdom, not without—forced and unwelcome as it might be to those of us going through it—a profound understanding of the human experience. . . . Parents with dying kids have insights into parenting and they are hard-won, forged through the prism of the hellish grief and helplessness and deeply committed love. These women had learned lessons not just about how to be a mother but how to be *human*." Finally, several writers wanted to spread awareness of certain problems, such as the high prevalence of Alzheimer's disease, the overwhelming burdens on caregivers, and medicine's emphasis on cure at any cost; some also called for social action. Those various motivations strongly influenced the way the authors constructed their accounts, further challenging any notion that they presented objective reality.[22]

The different chapters address the book's major themes. The first two chapters, "The Human Touch" and "Hope Became a Companion in Our Home," examine the issue of autonomy, asking questions such as, What kinds of information do dying people and families want? To what extent do both groups participate in practices of concealment? To what extent do they share in decisions about entering clinical trials? Chapter 3, "When Medicine Fails," asks, To what extent do dying people and their families view acceptance of the inevitable as a necessary ingredient of a good death? What are some of the virtues and uses of denial? What role do religion and spirituality play in helping people achieve acceptance? Chapter 4, "Caring by Kin," and chapter 5, "The Shadow Workforce," return to the topic of autonomy by focusing on dependency, an inescapable feature of human life. Both at home and in institutions, very sick people rely on relatives not only for medical and practical help but also to sustain dignity and self-worth. What barriers do those caregivers face? To what extent do such responsibilities undermine caregivers' own sense of autonomy? Chapter 6, "The Evolution of Hospice Care," analyzes how hospices have affected kin. Did the founders of the hospice movement understand the difficulties of moving death out of hospitals and nursing homes without compensating for all the services those institutions provide? To what extent have policymakers viewed the emphasis on home care primarily as a way to control costs? Are family members satisfied with the support hospices provide? What kinds of assistance are most important to them?

"God never gives you more than you can handle" is a familiar bromide. According to his daughter Anna, Sigmund Freud held a far darker view of the human predicament: "What one is able to bear is seldom what one must bear." This book is about people forced to contend with troubles that often seemed unendurable.[23]

1

"The Human Touch"

Defining the Good Doctor

"What did I expect from him?," psychiatrist Gordon Livingston asked rhetorically about the physician who had diagnosed his six-year-old son Lucas with leukemia in the late 1980s. Eight months earlier, Livingston's twenty-two-year-old son Andrew, a Swarthmore College student, had committed suicide. Now the father had to contemplate the loss of another child. Livingston acknowledged that Dr. Norton had delivered his news in a straightforward way. He had not concealed the seriousness of the disease by offering unrealistic hope or reassurance. As a doctor himself, Livingston understood that no one could make a prediction at such an early stage. But something was missing. "I realized that what I wanted was some form of understanding of what it was like for a father to face the news that his vibrantly healthy son, who a few hours ago seemed to have an inconsequential cold, carried with him a malignant disease that might kill him—and that it was now my job to convey that verdict to his mother and eleven-year-old sister. Our lives were being turned upside down. Whatever happened, we would never be the same."[1]

Livingston's experience reflected the changes that had occurred in medical care during the previous century. Livingston could accept as a matter of course that Dr. Norton would speak candidly, not only because Livingston was a physician, but also because doctors were far less likely than their predecessors to conceal critical information. At the same time, however, doctors were more likely to view disease solely as a biological phenomenon divorced from the context of individual lives. When Livingston first encountered Norton, few medical schools provided instruction about how to empathize with the suffering of patients and families and accompany them throughout the long course of a terminal chronic disease.

Truth Telling

Health professionals, ethicists, and scholars frequently debate whether doctors should reveal grim diagnoses and prognoses. Some argue that because concealment confers power, candor can help to equalize the relationship between doctors and patients. People who understand the gravity of their conditions are less likely to choose costly, aggressive, and often ineffective treatments at the end of life. Accurate prognostic information when death is inevitable enables people to make practical, spiritual, and emotional preparations. And secrecy may heighten the sense of shame and horror surrounding mortality; like a literal skeleton in the closet, death becomes too terrible even to be mentioned. Other commentators contend that bad medical news can shatter the sense of self, precipitate panic and despair, undermine the ability to cope, and even accelerate mortality.[2]

Nineteenth-century doctors refrained from making what the American Medical Association called "gloomy prognostications." The prominent physician Austin Flint explained that emotions exerted a powerful impact on disease outcome: "Undue solemnity, anxiety, and apprehension in the looks, manner, or words of a medical attendant on the sick are extremely unfortunate—they discourage patients, whereas, on the other hand, a cheerful mien, calmness of deportment, and verbal assurances, sometimes accomplish more than drugs."[3]

The growing gap between professional and lay knowledge at the turn of the twentieth century helped doctors conceal bad news. Although little had differentiated the ideas and practices of physicians from those of laypeople throughout much of the nineteenth century, physicians could claim unique competence by the early twentieth century. They alone had access to diagnostic tools, and they spoke a language few patients could comprehend. Because they had a better understanding of diseases as distinct entities in all patients, doctors also could more accurately predict the outcome. The few doctors who revealed cancer diagnoses exaggerated the promise of the therapies administered and denied evidence of recurrences.[4]

In the late 1950s, doctors began to question the tradition of concealment. Louis Lasagna, a professor at the Johns Hopkins School of Medicine, asserted that the physician "often avoid[s] telling patients or relatives about imminent death" because his "ego and peace of soul are apt to be assaulted by the knowledge that he is unable to alter the downhill course. He may feel uncomfortable and ill at ease; he may also be so busy that he is reluctant to take the time required to get to know the patient and the family well enough to do the job properly." Other doctors surveyed current practices. The most frequently cited study was by Donald Oken, who reported in 1961 that 90 percent of doctors still did not inform patients they had cancer. Some physicians used euphemisms, speaking of a "mass" or a "lesion," rather than a "neoplasm" or "cancer." A few asserted that a cancerous tumor was benign. When treatment was necessary, doctors gave just enough information to obtain compliance.[5]

But soon after Oken issued his report, various forces began to encourage greater openness. The first major sociological study of dying people in hospitals, conducted in the early 1960s by Barney G. Glaser and Anselm L. Strauss, analyzed four different "awareness contexts." Under conditions of closed awareness, patients did not know death was imminent, although nurses and doctors did. In the suspicion awareness context, patients suspected they were dying and tried to determine whether their suspicions were correct. In open awareness, both patients and staff freely acknowledged the approach of death. The fourth context, mutual pretense, existed when both patients and staff knew death was approaching but tried to pretend otherwise. Glaser and Strauss concluded that those different contexts determined the types of social interaction that would occur between dying people and hospital personnel.[6]

Elisabeth Kübler-Ross's 1969 book *On Death and Dying,* arguing that concealment intensified patients' sense of loneliness and isolation, reached a large popular audience. The hospice movement, launched in the 1970s, gave a high value to physician honesty. And the growing emphasis on autonomy in that decade prompted increasing arguments that patients and families had a right to know, even when the diagnosis was grim and the prognosis poor.[7]

Two memoirs demonstrate the impact of the culture of rights. Gerda Lerner was well on her way to becoming one of the most celebrated American historians in 1972 when her husband Carl,* a prominent film editor, was diagnosed with a malignant brain tumor. In 1958, at age thirty-eight, she had returned to school, earning a Columbia University PhD in history in 1966. By 1972 she had written two pathbreaking books and numerous

---

*I use first names only when two or more people under discussion have the same last name.

articles in women's history. That year she was a professor of history at Sarah Lawrence College, launching the first graduate program in women's history. With Carl's encouragement, Gerda continued her active professional life after his diagnosis, hiring helpers to provide much of the hands-on care. But she was often alone with Carl, and she monitored the care others provided, interacted frequently with his physicians, and made a variety of both medical and nonmedical decisions. *A Death of One's Own*, Gerda's narrative of Carl's illness and death, appeared in 1978.

Gerda recalled that the day after a doctor revealed that Carl's tumor was malignant, a nurse urged her to read Kübler-Ross's book and follow its injunction about speaking honestly. But Gerda consulted various experts who were unanimous in warning that Carl would suffer terrible harm if he knew his condition was hopeless. Against her better judgment, Lerner complied with their advice. "In retrospect I am sorry I did not follow my instinct and my convictions," she wrote. "It was bad advice I got and I believe it stemmed, unconsciously and though offered with the best of intentions, from a profound fear and denial of death." Her evasiveness not only clouded her relationship with Carl but also violated his autonomy: "The terminal patient has no time for subterfuge and denial. If he does not want to hear the truth, he will shut it out. But if he does want to hear it, who are we to keep it from him? It is his death, not ours. Every man and woman has the right to his or her own death."[8]

In the second case, a physician employed the language of rights. Joan Gould's book *Spirals: A Woman's Journey through Family Life* opened with an account of her learning in 1978 that her husband Martin, a litigation lawyer, had colon cancer. Joan urged the surgeon not to disclose the diagnosis to Martin because he had only a fifty-fifty chance of survival. "I feel my patients have a right to be informed," the surgeon replied.[9]

The push for greater openness occasionally extended to children. In 1978 Myra Bluebond-Langner published *Private Worlds of Dying Children*, a major anthropological study of terminally ill children ages three to nine. Drawing on the framework Glaser and Strauss had formulated a decade earlier, Bluebond-Langner concluded that dying children, their parents, and hospital staff operated under conditions of mutual pretense. Children with fatal diseases soon acquired information about their prognoses but assumed neither their parents nor hospital personnel knew. As death approached, children tried to distance themselves from both groups to guard their dangerous secret.[10]

That argument influenced at least one memoir writer. Terry Pringle, a copyeditor and writer, had just moved his family from Houston to Abilene, Texas, when he learned that his four-year-old son Eric had leukemia. Rushing to the local library, Pringle found the newly published *Private Worlds of Dying Children*. The book "reveals a larger view of children than the one I have," Pringle wrote. "I have never liked pretense and decide as I read that I will be whatever Eric needs. If he is dying and wants to discuss his condition openly, I will suspend my emotions and do just that."[11]

In 1979 a landmark study of physician practices appeared. Using Oken's questionnaire, Dennis H. Novack and colleagues reported that 97 percent of physicians informed patients they had cancer, a stunning reversal from 1961. Citing that research, numerous scholars have argued that the era of secrecy had ended.[12]

Recent evidence, however, points to a more tentative conclusion. Studies repeatedly report that although doctors are far more willing than their predecessors to disclose disturbing diagnoses, the great majority continue to hide grave prognoses. Memoirs published long after Novack's survey support that finding. Writers continually complained that after revealing cancer diagnoses, doctors concealed the seriousness of the disease or exaggerated the effectiveness of the treatments administered. Surgeons who removed malignant tumors reported that they had "gotten it all." As one irate adult daughter explained in 2010, "It only takes one residual cell to restart the nightmare, and the doctors can never know for sure whether they did in fact 'get it all.'" The same year a second daughter wrote that an oncologist had reassured her father-in-law that despite the late stage of his cancer, advanced age, and a heart condition, chemotherapy offered a significant chance of cure. Three days after his first cycle, he arrived in the emergency room, unable to eat or drink and suffering intense pain. A few weeks later, he was dead.[13]

Other writers charged that doctors avoided all discussion of disease outcome. Stan Mack was a cartoonist at the *Village Voice* when his partner Janet Bode, an author of books for teenagers, learned she had breast cancer. In his graphic memoir about Bode's diagnosis, treatment, and death, Mack noted that he had many frank conversations with the oncologist about treatment side effects when the disease returned in 1999. The doctor's discussion of the expected disease course, however, was "ambiguous." "How much improvement could we expect from the new chemo? What physiological changes should we prepare for and how should we handle them? Was she terminal and, if so, how much time did she have? Who was to tell us what we didn't know to ask?" Even when asked direct questions, many doctors hedged. Novelist Laurie Foos wrote that it "had been a battle to get the doctors to admit" that her father's cancer was incurable and his dialysis a form of palliative care.[14]

To be sure, the attitudes of patients and family members rarely were all of a piece. Despite the many complaints about physician secretiveness, relatives occasionally acknowledged that they did not always want to know the worst. Although Terry Pringle knew that his son was unlikely to get better, he felt tempted to slap his wife when she asked a doctor about the boy's chance of survival after a relapse. The response was "about five to ten percent." Mary Winfrey Trautmann lived in Whittier, California, with her husband and three daughters. In the 1970s she became active in the women's movement and in 1980 helped to found a small, independent, feminist press, which five years later published her memoir of her daughter Carol's illness and death from leukemia. Soon after learning the diagnosis, Mary Winfrey wrote, "I do not intend to become an authority on Carol's leukemia. Intuitively, I desire to keep all bitter informants at bay, to study no discouraging life expectancy charts or bleak percentages." Overhearing the doctor talk to her husband, Mary Winfrey learned several grim facts "almost against my will."[15]

Decades later, many memoir writers revealed similar attitudes. A publisher, editor, and journalist, Will Schwalbe recalled the many hours he had spent discussing books in hospital waiting rooms with his mother. A former director of admissions at Harvard, Mary Anne Schwalbe had worked with refugees for twenty years before she was diagnosed with pancreatic cancer in 2007 at age seventy-three. During the two years she battled the disease, she had numerous hospital admissions. Each time, her family frequently talked about her discharge date. "We never went near a discussion of a timetable beyond that," Will wrote, "how many more days, or weeks, or months, or years we might have with Mom—not just because it was impossible to know but because it was too painful." And Stanley Mack later wondered whether the responses of Janet Bode's doctor were as ambiguous as he had thought. "Or did we just refuse to consider the idea of death?"[16]

In addition, family members themselves employed various forms of secrecy. Some were relatively innocuous. For example, partners and spouses of people with AIDS frequently kept silent after seeing friends whose health had badly deteriorated or after reading notices of AIDS deaths. When relatives were privy to medical information that had been withheld from patients, however, the consequences of concealment could be more serious, as Gerda Lerner had discovered.

Face-to-face with their gravely ill relatives, some family members quailed at the prospect of speaking the truth. Philip Roth provided a uniquely eloquent description of a son's evasiveness. The doctor had told him that without extremely major surgery, his father would die from the tumor found on an MRI. But seeing his father "slumped down in a corner of the sofa waiting for the verdict," Philip could not bring himself to say the lines he had carefully rehearsed:

> I sat in the chair across from him, my heart pounding as though I were the one about to be told something terrible. "You have a serious problem," I began, "but it can be dealt with. You have a tumor in your head. Dr. Meyerson says that given the location, the chances are ninety-five percent that it's benign." I had intended, like Meyerson, to be candid and describe it as large, but I couldn't. That there was a tumor seemed enough for him to take in. Not that he had registered any shock as yet—he sat there emotionless, waiting for me to go on. "It's pressing on the facial nerve, and that's what's caused the paralysis." Meyerson had told me that it was wrapped *around* the facial nerve, but I couldn't say that either.[17]

If the memoirs suggest that both physicians and family members occasionally wavered in their commitment to honesty, however, medical secrecy dramatically diminished. By the time Gordon Livingston received the devastating news about his son Lucas, large numbers of doctors presented equally terrible information clearly and candidly.

Popular Medical Information

One reason doctors were able to conceal bad news so effectively for many years is that patients and families had few ways of obtaining medical information by themselves. Elaine Ipswitch and her husband Ronnie were living in Fillmore, a small southern California city in 1971, when their ten-year-old son Scott was diagnosed with Hodgkin's disease. Previously a telephone lineman, Ronnie was now co-owner of a shoe store. Assumptions about the parents' lack of education may partially explain the condescending treatment they received. When Elaine asked Scott's doctor to recommend something she could read, he replied, "There's some material in medical textbooks, but it's all so technical I don't think you'd get anything out of it." The following day, Ronnie asked another physician to tell them about the disease. Elaine wrote, "I never will forget that doctor sitting there and saying, 'Well, I'm trying to think how I can bring it down to a level you will understand.'" Elaine then consulted a third doctor, who "told us that the only meaningful information was in medical journals, but that by the time it was published, it was already obsolete because such strides were being made in treatment." Family members could look for announcements about recent breakthroughs in newspapers and magazines, but most articles were written in a triumphant style, omitting all qualifying statistics and thus fostering inflated expectations.[18]

Parents of children with leukemia had one other source of information. In 1964 the federal government issued *Childhood Leukemia: A Pamphlet for Parents*. The lead author, Dr. Stanford B. Friedman, made it clear that he had no intention of challenging medical control of information. Parents might find that pamphlet helpful because "some understanding of the disease [was] less frightening than ignorance and the unknown." But Friedman advised physicians to keep much information to themselves: "For instance, it is generally unwise to interpret the full medical implications of a falling white count in a child with leukemia, as most parents are not in the position to comprehend the many medical complexities and may inappropriately attempt to enter into the therapeutic decisions."[19]

Parents clearly wanted more. After her daughter's leukemia diagnosis in 1973, Mary Winfrey Trautmann complained that the material for parents was "certainly inadequate." Five years later, Terry Pringle dashed to the library because he found the publication distributed by the hospital too "brief." But change already had begun. One notable event was the publication of the first version of *Our Bodies, Ourselves* in 1971. Filled with detailed and easily accessible information, that manual as well as subsequent and greatly enlarged editions not only educated a generation of women about their health but also encouraged them to demand that doctors speak more honestly and share decision-making power. The consumer movement similarly promoted the democratization of medical information. A 1978 study reported that the *Readers' Guide* contained twice the number of citations to articles on health and illness it had had ten years earlier. Popular manuals on specific diseases lined bookstore shelves.[20]

Seriously ill children, too, occasionally had access to medical information. *You and Leukemia: A Day at a Time* was published in 1978, the year Terry Pringle's son was diagnosed. As one contemporary reviewer wrote, the book had an optimistic tone, but "the ultimate question—what happens if treatment doesn't work—is not ducked." With the help of that book, Pringle and his wife talked to their son about his illness. Pringle later explained, "The book illustrates blood in its normal state, in abnormal states where platelets and red cells and infection-fighting white cells are absent, and the resulting hemorrhage, anemia, and infection." As a result, "at the age of four, Eric is getting a significant education."[21]

With the coming of the World Wide Web, the amount of consumer medical information exploded. A 2003 survey found that half of adult Americans had searched for health information on the Internet. Reading and interpreting scans and tests remained the doctors' prerogative, but it became more difficult to hide diagnoses and prognoses once people could learn on their own about the symptoms, expected course, and life expectancies of different ailments.[22]

"A Common Sorrow"

If the spread of popular medical information helped to equalize relationships between physicians and both patients and family members, other forces rendered them more distant. Following contemporary medical beliefs, nineteenth-century doctors had valued personal connections to patients to reduce stress and gain critical knowledge. At the turn of the twentieth century, biological reductionism rendered irrelevant the patients' emotional and moral state, interaction with providers, and physical surroundings. Medical schools also encouraged students to shield themselves against patient suffering. The growing use of medical technology further separated physicians from patients. By the early years of the twenty-first century, it had become almost commonplace to complain that doctors' reliance on machinery to diagnose, treat, and monitor disease had reduced the importance of personal investigation of patients.[23]

Despite those developments, some memoir writers described doctors who conveyed painful information with warmth and solicitude. The naturalist and author Terry Tempest Williams was one. She wrote her memoir, *Refuge,* largely as a protest against the federal government's testing of nuclear weapons in the West, which she blamed for the many cases of breast cancer in her family. The book began with her mother's diagnosis of ovarian cancer and ended with her death five years later. Living close to her mother in Utah, Williams was intimately involved in her care. The doctor who told the mother she had a fatal disease was the obstetrician who had delivered two of her four babies. After giving her the X-ray results, he put his arm through hers and told her how sorry he was. He wished he had been able to give a more encouraging report. Later, when she was close to death, he "unfolds the truth to her like a red rose: petal by petal."[24]

Many more narratives, however, contained serious complaints. Large numbers of doctors were accused of fleeing after giving the diagnosis or providing it in inappropriate places. Terry Pringle remembered being escorted to "a cramped office room" by a hematologist "along with his ever present entourage of medical students" to hear what his son's tests had revealed. Although "Acute Lymphoblastic Leukemia has an explosive sound," Pringle wrote, he found himself "unsettled not by the sound of the name but by the meeting itself. The three students sit like bright-eyed evaluators for a game show, hoping we will prove to be suitable contestants." Stan Mack recalled how he and Janet Bode first heard she had breast cancer in 1994: "The surgeon met us in a busy and narrow corridor just off the main lobby. There, opposite the cashier's office, he gave us the bad news . . . and rushed off. His abruptness was so unnerving we could hardly absorb the diagnosis."[25]

Other criticisms were directed at the way doctors announced that death was inevitable. Rose Levit, a teacher in Novato, California, still was reeling from her husband's decision to leave the marriage and her older daughter's angry departure from home, when eleven-year-old Ellen was diagnosed with bone cancer in December 1970. Ellen's father, David, moved back to help care for her but made it clear he wanted a divorce. Jana, her older sister, returned off and on. When Ellen's disease continued to spread despite several months of treatment, the doctor suggested she consult a surgeon at a university hospital. After examining Ellen, the surgeon met with both parents. Rose later recalled that because he was too busy to find an empty room, they "stood in the corridor, while the surgeon explained in detached remote tones that given the site of Ellen's tumor, he could see no way of performing surgery." Even partial removal of the tumor would only accelerate metastasis. "It was like a death sentence," Rose wrote. "For me, hope of saving Ellen's life ended that day in October, during this hurried meeting in the hospital corridor."[26]

Like Gordon Livingston, Richard Lischer, a Duke University theology professor and a former Protestant clergyman, wrote about the loss of a son. He, too, demanded not just courtesy but also recognition of emotional and spiritual suffering. Adam Lischer was a lawyer in his early twenties, recently married and looking forward to the birth of his first child, when he learned his melanoma had returned. Richard attended most of the appointment. Later he wrote that the oncologist "spoke in perfectly constructed sentences with no syntactical breaks or interjections, as if he had diagrammed them before our meeting." The news was shattering: "We were plunging from a Stage 2 with a 70 percent chance of non-recurrence to a Stage 4 with a 15 percent chance of *response to treatment* . . . with absolutely no talk of cure, no Stage 5, no reasonable prospects for effective treatment, and no mention of survival." Richard was acutely aware of what was missing: "We would have welcomed the human touch—some crumb of acknowledgement that, even though he was the doctor and our son was the patient, we were at least capable, all of us, of a common sorrow, no matter how differently it might be expressed."[27]

Memoir writers also criticized physician behavior when death drew close. A few accused doctors of withdrawing to avoid acknowledging that the possibility of a cure had ended. Stan Mack wrote that after Jane Bode tried various types of chemotherapy without success, her oncologist suggested they get together to evaluate whether to discontinue therapy. But when Bode's condition sharply deteriorated, Mack was unable to contact the doctor for weeks despite several attempts by both phone and e-mail. Mack was aware that troubles in the oncologist's life partly explained her silence; she did, however, respond immediately when another doctor called on Bode's behalf. In a brief phone conversation, the oncologist recommended that Bode enroll in hospice. She never found time for the extensive discussion Bode and Mack had been led to expect.[28]

Alan Shapiro's brother-in-law also needed the intervention of another doctor to speak to an oncologist at a critical juncture. Alan was a poet and professor of English at the University of North Carolina, Chapel Hill. His sister Beth was a librarian at Rice University and the mother of a young child. The two siblings were very close, especially after their parents had disowned Beth for marrying an African American man. She had received extensive therapy for breast cancer, first a mastectomy, chemotherapy, radiation, and a stem cell transplant, and then, after a recurrence, additional rounds of chemotherapy. But when she reported headaches, dizziness, and backaches in 1995, the doctor ordered a spinal tap to help reassess the therapeutic plan. Arriving for a visit, Alan learned that Beth's husband Russ "had been calling the oncologist all week to find out what, if anything, the spinal tap had revealed. But the doctor hadn't called him back. He was tired of waiting, tired of being put on hold, tired of not knowing." In desperation, Russ asked a cardiologist friend to try to make contact. Less than a minute after the cardiologist left a message, the oncologist phoned back, confirming what her family had begun to suspect. Treatment would now be futile. Soon after that conversation, the family transferred Beth to a hospice facility.[29]

Two weeks later, the oncologist again disappointed. Early one morning, Alan found him standing beside Beth's bed. She was awake, waiting for the doctor to speak. After a long silence, he said, " 'Let's see what they have you on.' And he pulled out from beneath her pillow the . . . morphine pump, the thread-thin IV tube running from it to her shoulder. 'Uh-huh,' he said, 'very good.' Then he checked her chart and after another moment said, 'So.' Then more silence. Then his beeper went off. He glanced at it, said he had to go, but that he'd be back soon in a day or so to see how she was doing." That was the last time they saw him.[30]

Gordon Livingston had agreed with the recommendation that his son receive a bone marrow transplant. As a result, he blamed himself as well as the oncologist, when the treatment ended in disaster. Nevertheless, the father accused Dr. Norton of betrayal. A week after Lucas's death, Livingston decided the doctor should read the journal Livingston had kept throughout the ordeal. "I hope he learns something from it—about what such an experience is like for the family of a dying child," Livingston wrote. "It still bothers us that he left on a . . . junket to Saudi Arabia on the day before Lucas died. Since then, not a word have we heard from him." Although two nurses and a nephrologist attended the funeral, Norton never arrived. Sending Norton a copy of the diary a few days later, Livingston enclosed a cover letter that read in part, "While I do not hold you responsible for what has happened to us, I think you will understand why I am sorry I ever met you."[31]

Medical Residents

Residents are recent medical school graduates who are receiving additional training, typically by working in hospitals. Although the memoir writers leveled a wide assortment of criticisms at the medical profession as a whole, they singled out residents for special condemnation. Most relatives had spent long periods of time in hospitals, where residents delivered the bulk of care. Virtually no author had anything good to say about them.

Soon after their twenty-year-old son told Marcia Friedman and her husband Lieb that he had a malignant brain tumor in 1972, they closed their Santa Barbara real estate practice and moved to West Los Angeles, close to the UCLA Medical Center, where Josh was to receive care. Marcia recalled that several residents ignored his serious symptoms after surgery. A year later he was dying and needed pain medication that could not be administered at home. After his parents brought him back to the hospital, he had to wait more than an hour before a resident saw him. Then another hour elapsed while the resident proceeded to conduct a lengthy examination. Because Josh was writhing on the bed and begging for help, Marcia finally "turned to that incredibly insensitive, pompous fool costumed to play the role of healer and insisted that he get some relief to Josh." The resident not only refused but ordered the parents out of the room. They reluctantly complied.[32]

The sportswriter Frank Deford charged the resident who cared for his daughter with both incompetence and deceit. Alex had been diagnosed with cystic fibrosis at age one. In November 1979 she was eight and near the end of her life. Having just spent two weeks in Yale–New Haven Hospital, she was looking forward to going home when her lung suddenly collapsed. She immediately knew what had happened. "But the young resident on the floor seemed threatened that an eight-year-old could be usurping his diagnostic responsibility," Deford wrote. "He told Alex she was wrong, her lung had not collapsed. Not only that, he refused to give her X rays." Soon afterward, Alex's mother and grandmother came for a visit. After listening to Alex, they urged the resident to summon her physician, Dr. Dolan. The resident lied, claiming that he already had called Dr. Dolan and that he would be in shortly.[33]

An adult daughter gave an equally horrific report about care in a county hospital in 1993. After her mother was diagnosed with terminal esophageal cancer, Hillary Johnson, an author and journalist, moved from New York to Minneapolis to provide care. When her mother suffered excruciating pain after a nurse dislodged the feeding tube, a resident concluded she was having a heart attack and transferred her to a cardiac unit. There Hillary fought with another resident who decided the mother needed major surgery. Later, yet another resident made disastrous mistakes trying to insert a tracheotomy tube.[34]

Family members occasionally protested. Writing in the 1980s, Jacquie Gordon couched her story in the language of rights. She had been married to puppeteer Jerry Nelson (later well known for his work with the Muppets on *Sesame Street*) when their daughter Christine was born. But Gordon and Nelson soon separated, and the mother raised the girl largely on her own. Diagnosed with cystic fibrosis at a young age, Christine was eight when she was hospitalized with viral pneumonia in 1969. Remembering an earlier experience with needles, Christine became terrified when a resident announced he was about to start intravenous antibiotics. Gordon thus promised to stay by her side and hold her hand. The doctor barred the mother's entry to the treatment room. After standing outside, listening to her daughter's screams, Gordon burst into the room, demanding that the resident find another doctor. "The resident and his staff stared at me," she wrote.

> I didn't move. Chris didn't move. What was going to happen? Then the resident turned to one of the nurses and said in a blasé tone, "Go get Dr. Whitcomb. He's good at this." And just like that, without a word to me, the nurse left to get him. I was furious and turned to the resident.
>
> "Why didn't you do that before?"
>
> "I'm sorry. Her veins are very difficult."
>
> "Her veins are nothing of the kind." But suddenly I understood. I could have stopped him at any time. I could have insisted they let me in. This was a teaching hospital. He was a student. I could have refused to let him touch her. I hadn't known I had any rights at all, but I knew now.[35]

But protest was rarely so successful. Frank Deford complained in a letter to Yale–New Haven Hospital, and although he received nice replies from some doctors, he had no confidence that he had changed hospital policy. Hillary Johnson later discovered that the cardiac resident with whom she had fought had included with his case notes a long addendum about her difficult behavior.[36]

Conclusion

Here it is especially important to remember the subjectivity of memoirs. Because the research for this chapter included neither observation of medical encounters nor interviews with doctors, it is impossible to establish the validity of the memoirs' retrospective accounts. Although insecurity may have made some residents as arrogant and incompetent as those accounts suggest, the harshness of the comments suggests other forces were at work as well. Perhaps family members found it easier to direct their rage toward residents, whose rotations lasted only a few months, than at the physicians who remained on the case for years. Family members who hated their dependency on the medical establishment may have been especially irate when they found themselves relying on doctors who were, in many cases, younger than themselves. And with the lives of loved ones hanging in the balance, the writers could not bear the thought that anyone other than the most distinguished doctor would read test results, make therapy decisions, and administer treatment.

The heightened emotions family members brought to each physician encounter also may have led them to misinterpret or forget some of what even established doctors said. Desperate for a reason to hope, some may not even have heard information about survival rates. Terry Pringle acknowledged that parents often projected their anger at the disease onto the physician who could not deliver a cure. A few other memoir writers offered excuses for the impersonality physicians displayed. Young, inexperienced doctors were overwhelmed by the terrifying situations they could not control. Older physicians had cared for too many fatally ill patients to continue to treat each as a unique individual. AIDS doctors had to shield themselves emotionally from the relentless march of death they witnessed. Doctors critical of their profession have noted other factors as well—the doctrine of detached concern inculcated during medical training and pressures from an increasingly intolerable workload.[37]

In this chapter, two fathers of dying sons demanded not only that doctors speak honestly and considerately but also that they recognize the anguish of both dying individuals and their families, express empathy, and travel with them during the long road to death. Chapter 6 argues that the founders of hospices in the 1970s and 1980s expected the staff to offer such services, attending to emotional and spiritual suffering, not just physical pain. We will see, however, that some memoir writers rejected that help, seeking practical and medical assistance alone.

2

"Hope Became a Companion in Our Home"

Enrolling in Clinical Trials

"How to reconcile the reality of human mortality with the reigning assumption in the rich world that every disease must have a cure, if not now then sometime in the future?" asks writer David Rieff in his memoir of the illness and death of his mother, Susan Sontag. "The logic of the former is the acceptance of death. But the logic of the latter is that death is somehow a mistake, and that someday that mistake will be rectified." For Sontag, as for large numbers of others, a search for an experimental treatment provided the way to cling to the second belief.[1]

After the end of World War II, people with terminal disease increasingly received experimental therapies, especially for cancer. By the 1970s, large numbers of people entered clinical trials after conventional therapies failed. Twenty years later, US cancer research centers reported that they had enough clinical trials to enable every advanced cancer patient to enter one. Recent studies conclude that the benefits of participation in that research rarely outweigh the risks for people near the end of life, that the purpose of trials is to help future patients, not present ones, and that investigators often encourage patients and family members to confuse research and treatment. Nevertheless, oncologists today commonly consider referral to a clinical study an integral part of the care of people with advanced, incurable cancer.[2]

Dramatic changes in public perception of medical research have accompanied its expansion. America's victory in World War II, abetted by the development of penicillin, radar, and the atomic bomb, generated unprecedented optimism about the entire scientific enterprise throughout the late 1940s and 1950s. The war "taught one lesson of incalculable importance," the *Women's Home Companion* wrote in 1946. "The lesson: that with unlimited money to spend we can buy the answers to almost any scientific problem." Both private and public funding for medical research soared. At one major university-affiliated hospital, for example, the money for research grew from $500,000 in 1945 to $8 million in 1965, a 2,000 percent increase.[3]

But optimism about medical science did not last. Beginning in the late 1960s, a wide variety of social movements inspired distrust of all established authorities, including physicians. Patients increasingly demanded information about diseases and treatment options and participation in medical decision making. And a growing number of reports revealed that the interests of researchers and patients commonly diverged and that joining a study could endanger as well as extend life.

Although many family narratives use the terms "experimental treatment" and "clinical trial" imprecisely, they do have clear definitions. Experimental treatments are therapies that are not yet proven by the medical community as safe and effective. Clinical trials are studies conducted on humans to compare experimental therapies with those already approved. Since the 1950s, medicine has accepted the randomized control trial as the gold standard; large numbers of studies, however, have departed from that model. In all studies, physicians must adhere to a protocol and cannot make decisions on the basis of individual health needs. Several memoirs discussed experimental treatments without indicating whether or not they were being tested in clinical trials. In what follows, I use the terms "experimental treatment" and "clinical trial" as they appear in the different family narratives.[4]

In Harry M. Marks's classic history of medical experimentation in the United States, he writes, "I have yet to encounter a source that would tell me much about patients, other than as researchers imagined them." The patients chronicled in the family memoirs used in this study can hardly be considered typical. Disproportionately affluent and well educated, they were more likely than others to gain access to experimental interventions, acquire medical expertise, and challenge physician authority. Nevertheless, the narratives help to fill the void Marks highlighted.[5]

Death Be Not Proud

To highlight how shifting attitudes toward medicine affected the response of patients and their families to clinical studies, it is important to begin with the postwar period, the apogee of popular faith in medical research. The June 27, 1949, issue of *Time* magazine epitomizes the widespread excitement surrounding the postwar cancer research industry. To one side of the cover was a drawing of a sword, symbolizing the American

Cancer Society, slashing through a crab. The rest of the cover was devoted to a picture of a grave but confident-looking Dr. Cornelius P. Rhoads, the director of both New York's Memorial Hospital for Cancer and Allied Diseases and the Sloan-Kettering Institute, established in 1945 as the nation's first cancer research institute. A former army officer, Rhoads had served during World War II as chief of the army's Chemical Warfare Unit, where he had been involved in experiments on mustard gas, a chemical weapon, and accidentally discovered that it might retard cancer cells. Now he argued that the scientists under his direction were fighting to destroy "an army of invaders of the body," using "atomic, chemical and biological means." Chemotherapy, increasingly Sloan-Kettering's focus, aroused even more interest because it was a systemic, rather than a local, treatment and thus could have far more effect on metastasized disease. Rhoads anticipated that drugs would be able to play the same role in cancer treatment that antibiotics performed in the cure of infectious disease. In 1953 Congress awarded the National Cancer Institute $3 million to test various chemotherapeutic drugs; and by 1958 scientists at various institutions annually screened tens of thousands of compounds.[6]

At a time of such widespread enthusiasm about the research enterprise, it seemed easy to leave ethical decisions to investigators' discretion. The 1947 Nuremberg Code that emerged from the Doctors' Trial in Nuremberg, Germany, enunciated a set of principles for the conduct of ethical research. The most important was that researchers engage in a process known as "informed consent," whereby they provide information about the study to potential human subjects and request their participation. Most American researchers, however, ignored the code, assuming that the work conducted in their laboratories bore no resemblance to the atrocities committed in concentration camps. The small number of investigators who heeded the informed consent provision believed it applied only to healthy volunteers, not to sick patients.[7]

Widespread paternalism in health care undoubtedly enhanced researchers' ability to convince parents that their dying children should participate in clinical trials. We have seen that throughout the 1950s and 1960s, few doctors disclosed cancer diagnoses. They also made major treatment decisions without consulting patients or families. Two doctors wrote in 1955 that "because of the considerable anxiety which parents of a child with a malignant disorder face," it was especially "undesirable to add to this anxiety by leaving decisions concerning treatment to them." A pediatrician at Children's Hospital, Boston, the site of many clinical trials, was more emphatic. "I make it very clear to parents of children with fatal diseases," he wrote in 1964, "that they are not going to be doctors." "I make certain that they know that the medical management must be firmly fixed in our hands as the physicians" and "that as far as decisions on what to do are concerned, the choice will be ours."[8]

But if parents of children with cancer had little autonomy, they often had their own reasons for seeking experimental treatments. Many had been told that their child would die very soon without therapy. In the absence of standard, effective treatments, desperate parents assumed they had no choice but to hunt for experimental ones. Faith in the march of medical progress enabled parents to believe the next breakthrough might miraculously cure their child. And by aligning themselves with medical research, parents were able to infuse their experiences with meaning, viewing themselves and their offspring as part of a larger whole. Even if the child ultimately died, they would have made an important contribution to the lives of those who followed.

The most famous postwar narrative by the parent of a child with cancer was John Gunther's *Death Be Not Proud*, describing the fifteen-month struggle of his seventeen-year-old son Johnny with a malignant brain tumor. Published in 1949, the year *Time* celebrated the triumphs of the cancer research industry, the book expressed the same confidence in medical science. "The thought never left us," Gunther wrote, "that if only we could defer somehow what everybody said was inevitable, if only we could stave off Death for a few weeks or months, something totally new might turn up." Well known as a journalist and the author of the *Inside* books about many countries, John Gunther was able to contact some of the most distinguished physicians in the country. By the end, he and his ex-wife Frances Gunther had consulted thirty-seven doctors.[9]

In addition to asking a wide array of doctors for advice, the parents relied on the two sources of medical information then available to the public. John "prodded [sic] through several texts full of the frightful jargon of medical writers," and both parents searched newspapers for the announcement of a medical breakthrough that might save their son. "One morning Frances found an item in the Sunday *Times* . . . describing some remarkable amelioration of tumors—not brain tumors, but just tumors—caused by intravenous dosages of mustard gas." John noted that none of his "eminent correspondents had so much as mentioned it. But there it was plain as day in the *New York Times*." Once again the Gunthers took advantage of their special connections. The family physician got in touch with Dr. Rhoads, and Gunther finally made contact with Dr. Joseph Burchenal, then a "young scientist with a fine war record," who directed the mustard gas experiments at Memorial Hospital. Within twenty-four hours of that meeting, Gunther witnessed "the first injection of mustard gas ever given at the Medical Center [Columbia-Presbyterian Hospital]," where Johnny received treatment. "It was all so impromptu and urgent" that the father "carried the precious, frightfully poisonous stuff from one hospital to the other." Although Johnny died soon afterward, Gunther's faith in medical science remained strong. He noted that he donated his profits from the book to cancer research in the hope that other young men could avoid his son's terrible fate. *Death Be Not Proud* rapidly became a best seller, and condensed versions appeared in popular magazines.[10]

Eric Lund's Cancer Treatment

Doris Lund's *Eric* was another best-selling memoir about a son's battle with cancer, but it described events that occurred in a very different context. By the time Eric Lund was diagnosed with leukemia in 1967, the public had received some of the first accounts of abuses in medical research. In 1957 the media reported that thousands of women in Europe, Canada, and to a far lesser extent the United States had delivered babies with serious birth defects as a result of taking the sedative thalidomide. Nine years later, a widely circulated article by Harvard researcher Henry K. Beecher in the *New England Journal of Medicine* documented twenty-two cases in which investigators had placed human subjects at risk without their knowledge or consent. A study conducted under the direction of Chester Southam, a medical school professor and cancer researcher, had injected live cancer cells into elderly patients with dementia at New York's Jewish Chronic Disease Hospital. Doris Lund's account of experimental treatments, however, was overwhelmingly positive.[11]

Doris Lund was already a published writer when she received the doctor's phone call that transformed the world she had known. Eric was then seventeen, an avid athlete, and looking forward to his freshman year at the University of Connecticut. As in *Death Be Not Proud*, a mother's discovery of a newspaper article altered the course of treatment. Four months after Eric began therapy from a local physician, Doris suddenly spotted a startling headline: "New Drug Offers Best Hope for Control of Leukemia." For the first time, she heard of a medication called asparaginase. Doris assumed that the news item was in part a public relations release, but she grew increasingly excited as she read, "Scientists cautiously predict that the new drug, which works on a completely different principle from the usual antileukemic drugs, offers new hope not only for control of the disease, but possibly for an eventual cure." Previous triumphs in the field of leukemia may have intensified her enthusiasm. By the mid-1960s, advances in chemotherapeutic treatments had successfully extended the lives of many young victims of the disease, suggesting that the hopes invested in postwar medical science might soon be realized. Doris understood that asparaginase was still experimental, supplies were extremely limited, and the cost per patient topped three hundred thousand dollars, an astronomical price in 1967. Nevertheless, she and her husband vowed that Eric would be one of the lucky few. Phoning the local oncologist the next morning, the parents learned he was both a friend and neighbor of Dr. Joseph Burchenal, the doctor whom John Gunther had consulted twenty years earlier. Now director of clinical investigation at Sloan-Kettering Institute, Burchenal was the man responsible for the promising breakthrough.[12]

Doris previously had hurried past the complex that included Memorial Hospital and the Sloan-Kettering Institute, assuming that the name meant death. But when she brought Eric for an appointment with Burchenal, the letters engraved on the side of the building filled her with hope. Although the doctor told Eric he would have to wait to obtain asparaginase, Doris felt far more secure after the appointment: "We were connected now to the center where the problem was being fought at every level with the strongest, most effective weapons in the world."[13]

When Burchenal finally decided Eric needed asparaginase, he entered the Ewing Pavilion (previously called Ewing Hospital), a tall, red-brick building contiguous to both Memorial Hospital and the Sloan-Kettering Institute. Ewing was one of two new three-hundred-bed New York City cancer hospitals that opened in the summer of 1950. Memorial and Sloan-Kettering donated the land and appointed the medical staff. The city paid construction costs and assumed responsibility for administrative, clerical, nursing, and maintenance personnel. Publicity surrounding the hospital emphasized that, for the first time, poor patients would have access to the best-trained physicians and state-of-the art treatments. Although the Lunds were not poor, they were freelance workers and had no health insurance. As a result, they already had found the cost of Eric's treatment extremely burdensome. So far, however, he had needed only the simplest and cheapest drugs; the price of the new medications he now would receive was much steeper. Doris thus was grateful that Eric "came under the protective umbrella of CRF, or Clinical Research Facility," which meant that the federal government paid for his care.[14]

What neither Lund nor the contemporary media noted was that the federal government's financial protection came at a price. Cornelius Rhoads, Ewing's director, stressed that the hospital was "originally built for research." In relying on low-income people as human subjects in medical experiments, Ewing followed a common practice. A committee established by President Bill Clinton to investigate human radiation experiments funded by the federal government in the postwar period later wrote that one researcher had provided "a frank description of a quid pro quo rationale that was probably quite common in justifying the use of poor patients in medical research: 'We were taking care of them, and felt we had a right to get some return from them, since it wouldn't be in professional fees and since our taxes were paying for their hospital beds.'" Although the extant records do not enable us to determine to what extent Ewing's research mission influenced Eric Lund's treatment, the New York City commissioner of hospitals reported that Ewing patients were "the focal point of the Sloan-Kettering Institute laboratory program of cancer research." It is thus highly likely that the drugs administered to Eric differed from those he would have received as a paying patient at Memorial.[15]

Eric drew support from many sources as he battled both the disease and the terrible consequences of his therapy. He developed a close rapport with Dr. Monroe Dowling, the chief of Memorial's Hematology Clinic. Burchenal expressed deep affection for Eric. Toward the end of his life, Eric established a romantic relationship with a private-duty nurse named Mary Lou. And he and the other patients forged a tight community. "There was no generation gap," Doris explained. "All the other gaps of race, color, religion, or country also tended to disappear in the face of the great common enemy—cancer. . . . As in a shipwreck or other large-scale disaster, when life came down to the basics, the things that counted were bravery, humor and the will to live." Sociologist Renée C. Fox found an equally close set of relationships on the ward she studied in the 1950s. The patients all suffered from terminal metabolic diseases and had agreed to become research subjects. "One of the primary ways in which the men . . . came to terms with their problems and stresses," Fox wrote, "was by deeply committing themselves to one another, and to the ward community which had emerged from the predicament they shared."[16]

Although the patients on Eric's floor went home during remissions, they frequently returned to the same ward and remained there for long periods of time. But death constantly disrupted the group. The first time a patient died in Eric's room, his mother was surprised to see no figure on the stretcher pushed by an orderly. "I didn't know then that the body was hidden on a shelf underneath," she wrote. "I hadn't yet learned that the dead vanish tactfully at Memorial. There are too many of them for anyone to bear."[17]

As the drugs given to Eric became more toxic and less effective, Doris praised the doctors' refusal to surrender. "They keep trying things as long as there's the slightest chance," she wrote. Such a fight to the end probably was not unusual. A few years before Eric's diagnosis, Dr. Rudolf Toch, a prominent cancer investigator, had stressed the special responsibilities of cancer research centers. When doctors know of nothing more to do to produce another remission in a child, and "death becomes inevitable," Toch wrote, they must ask how much they are "going to do with this youngster." Doctors in the community might turn to "supportive measures" (what we now would call "palliative care"), especially when children were suffering intense pain. In major research centers, however, scientific progress took priority over patient care. Doctors in those settings had the "obligation of exploring new ways of doing things" and thus had to use "new and untried agents of some promise." The final stage of life represented "a time of learning as well as of helping." "Morally," Toch conceded, "one would never use anything that does not hold some measure of promise." But he set a very low bar for that promise: "The nature of tumor chemotherapy is that you cannot predict; all the animal studies, all the preliminary tests do not predict what man will do with a given compound."[18]

Eric apparently shared his mother's abiding faith in medical science. Just after learning that one of his remissions had ended, he participated in a hospital seminar for oncology nurses. When asked whether he thought patients on the verge of death should be encouraged to face hard reality, he drew on his own experience:

> I could look to the future and say I'm running out of drugs. I'm becoming resistant to certain chemicals. My therapy has gone completely to hell. Maybe I should forget about the future. But there are doctors working across the street at Sloan-Kettering Institute. Doctors are working around the world who are, at the same time I'm running out of things, perfecting new things. So it's a questionable thing, as far as a doctor or a nurse dealing with somebody's denial of the disease. You might say the patient doesn't accept the fact that he's going to die. Well, in a lot of cases, it's questionable whether somebody's going to die or not.[19]

Soon after that seminar, Eric's doctors acknowledged they had only one more drug to try. That medication produced such unremitting nausea that Eric could barely eat for five weeks, lost forty pounds, and became unconscious. Now Dr. Dowling called a family conference. Because Eric was in kidney failure, Dowling was considering dialysis. Like most other doctors at the time, he stressed that he alone would make the final decision, but he wanted to know what family members thought. As Eric's parents, siblings, and girlfriend offered their opinions, the mother noticed Dr. Burchenal standing in the doorway and asked what more he had to offer if the dialysis succeeded. In her comments on his answer, she revealed her only discomfort with his aggressive approach. Burchenal responded, "Well . . . we have VP-Sixteen. It's quite effective with mice, and we've also had some interesting results with several humans." Overhearing Eric's girlfriend Mary Lou murmur "Jesus!" Doris thought: "We had already proved many times that Eric was not a mouse. And 'interesting results,' if they involved one more day of nausea, were not enough. Eric had come to the end of his will." Although "nobody wants to play God," it was time to "let him go." But the family was divided, and Dowling proceeded. Eric never regained consciousness and died a few days later.[20]

Like John Gunther, Doris Lund derived solace from the knowledge that her child had left an important legacy. The book ends with her husband Sidney giving blood in Memorial's Donor Room eighteen months after Eric's death. Doris imagined Sidney's blood flowing into another patient's veins, "perhaps stopping a hemorrhage, perhaps making it possible for him to walk in the world again." And one day, she was convinced, someone "was going to walk out of there cured and not have to go back." Although Doris "might not be around to see it," she was "connected just the same. And Eric would be part of that victory." We can only speculate about whether she would have written so positively about the research enterprise had she suspected that at least some of the drugs administered to her son had served the investigators' interests rather than his.[21]

Cancer Research in the 1970s

Eric Lund died in 1971, the year President Nixon signed the National Cancer Act, providing for a vast infusion of funds into cancer research and raising new expectations about the conquest of the nation's most fearsome affliction. The following year, however, a new shadow spread over medical research. Although the US Public Health Service had been conducting the Tuskegee Syphilis Study for forty years, the public did not learn about it until 1972. The study participants were poor African American men, who were neither told they had syphilis nor offered treatment, even after penicillin became widely used in the 1940s. Although thirteen reports of the study had appeared in major medical journals, none had received much attention. The 1972 exposé by the Associated Press, however, generated widespread outrage.[22]

Partly in response to that scandal, the federal government began to institute a regulatory system for research involving human subjects. At the heart of the new regime was the requirement that investigators obtain informed consent from patients participating in federally funded research. Newly established institutional review boards (IRBs) were entrusted with responsibility for enforcing compliance. Numerous studies have found that few patients read informed consent forms, that many of those who do read them fail to understand the researchers' intent, and that IRBs provide an inadequate bulwark against research abuse. Nevertheless, the regulations made it clear that the government and universities no longer would defer automatically to investigators' judgment about what constituted ethical practice.[23]

If revelations about research abuse spurred the government to action, however, they appear to have had little impact on many patients and family members. Most narratives of individuals diagnosed in the 1970s reflected the hopes inspired by the war on cancer rather than any fears aroused by media reports of past abuses. One explanation may lie in what bioethicists call the "therapeutic misconception," the widespread belief that treatment decisions for research subjects are based solely on their individual health needs. In fact, because the goal of clinical trials is scientific advancement, research needs take priority. Although people with low educational levels are more prone than others to misunderstand the purpose of clinical studies, well-educated patients are not exempt.[24]

In addition, the media focused primarily on incidents in which participants had been healthy when the studies began; in the memoirs, urgent need generated a search for experimental trials. And most studies that aroused condemnation had relied overwhelmingly on members of disadvantaged groups, including poor people, members of ethnic and minority groups, prisoners, and inmates of institutions for mentally retarded people. The predominantly privileged people chronicled in the memoirs may have assumed they had little in common with those populations. Historian Vanessa Northington Gamble wrote that the Tuskegee study "predisposed many African Americans to distrust medical and public health authorities and . . . led to critically low Black participation in clinical trials." As Gamble explained, the study had such a powerful effect because it meshed with the historical memory of the abuse of slave bodies in medical experimentation as well as with the current experience of African Americans in the health care system. It is thus striking that none of the mostly white authors of the narratives used in this chapter mentioned Tuskegee.[25]

Soon after Rose Levit's daughter Ellen began treatment for bone cancer in a hospital in a small northern California city, her father searched for new therapies and possible research breakthroughs, finally contacting a San Francisco hospital physician who described an experimental therapy in immunology under the direction of Dr. Al Lorin. Lorin, in turn, spoke enthusiastically about the transfer factor, which involved using a substance prepared from the white cells of the blood of a family member to try to boost the patient's ability to fight the disease. Although Ellen's parents understood that the prospect of recovery was remote, they grasped that opportunity. "At least now we were being given a chance to fight the cancer," Rose explained. "Even if we lost, as we were carefully warned would probably happen, at last we would fight." While continuing the radiation, Ellen began to receive monthly injections of the transfer factor from her father's blood. "Hope became a companion in our home that spring," Rose recalled.[26]

Rose seems to have had little doubt that the interests of medical science and those of her daughter coincided and that Lorin viewed Ellen as a person as well as a research subject. When Ellen's appetite and weight increased, "Dr. Lorin spoke triumphantly of the increase in 'rosette count' in Ellen's blood samples, a sign that her resistance was increasing. He carefully documented his research. We knew we were breaking ground and we dared to hope that Ellen would get well." When her weight and energy level again declined, Dr. Lorin began another innovative therapy, this time inoculating her with BCG, a drug used in Paris and a few other cancer centers. Despite his efforts, however, the tumor soon metastasized to the lung, and Ellen's life became engulfed in crushing pain. Lorin realized they had reached a crossroads. "It was important to his research to find out how long [his treatment] could be maintained," Rose wrote. "He believed that in carrying on his research he was also prolonging Ellen's life." But he acknowledged the possibility that his therapies might exacerbate her suffering. The decision was Ellen's to make. If she discontinued treatment, Lorin would provide pain medication to ease her final days. But he clearly hoped she would make a different choice. Seeking to encourage Rose and Ellen to identify with his research, he took them on a tour of his new laboratory. "With pride, he showed us the new equipment being purchased by the hospital. He talked of plans for computerized processes, which would diagnose cancer before it became the terrible life-devouring monster it now was." Although Ellen decided to continue her therapy, it proved ineffective and she died soon after it began.[27]

Long after Marcia Friedman urged her son to participate in a research study, she bitterly regretted having done so. At the time she had assumed she had no alternative. After her son Josh's disastrous surgery for brain cancer, however, she had ample reason to distrust the medical profession. The operation severely damaged his intellectual capabilities. Subsequently, they learned it probably had caused the tumor to metastasize. Nevertheless, when the oncologist suggested that he begin an experimental course of chemotherapy, Marcia could not "slough off almost half a century of indoctrination about the infallibility of doctors." True, the doctor acknowledged that the treatment could only retard the spread of the disease, not cure it. And Josh was decidedly unenthusiastic. "But I wanted my son to live," the mother later explained. "Although I knew he was not going to live, I tried to fool myself, to convince myself that this new physical torment would be helpful." The side effects of the first round of treatment were even worse than anticipated, and Josh returned for a second round only under pressure from his parents. This time the side effects were still more horrific. "Something in the chemical had caused a strange and frightening upset in his brain. He hallucinated and screamed in terror." His parents finally suspended the treatment and took him home to die.[28]

Experimental chemotherapy was not the only nonconventional therapy available for people with advanced cancer. By 1977, approximately six hundred bone marrow grafts had taken place. Although the procedure remained mired in difficulties, recommendations that patients undergo such transplantation occasionally provided a flicker of hope to them and their families. The local hematologist who diagnosed Mary Winfrey Trautmann's daughter Carol with leukemia in 1973 urged the mother to apply to the City of Hope, a major cancer center in Duarte, California, twenty miles east of Los Angeles. "If they are studying her particular kind of leukemia," the doctor was quoted as saying, "they may accept her as a patient." Carol must have satisfied the eligibility criteria, because she soon entered the hospital. If Mary Winfrey had any concerns about her daughter's participation in research studies, she did not mention them.[29]

The mother's memoir traced Carol's growing despondency and fury as she realized her chance of recovery was slim despite the increasingly aggressive therapy she endured. The possibility of a bone marrow transplant, however, cheered her, and she began to imagine undergoing the procedure with a friend, another girl on the ward. Her parents were equally enthusiastic, although the doctor warned that transplantation was still an experimental method and rarely had been tried, the bone marrow used in the graft would have to be completely compatible, and Carol's sisters, the most likely donors, would have to have their blood and lymphatic systems tested. The results of the blood tissue tests arrived the day after Christmas. "With great bitterness," Mary Winfrey underlined the date in her diary: "December 26, 1974. No go, no match, no donor."[30]

The same blow struck Elaine Ipswitch at L. A. Children's hospital, where her son Scott began treatment for Hodgkin's disease in 1971. Easily intimidated by the hospital staff, she became especially dependent on the other parents she met in the waiting room. A particular source of comfort was a woman named Joanne, whose son Richard became one of Scott's first roommates. "It was good to have someone to talk with and learn that

I was not the only one who found this hospital world uncomfortable and bewildering," Elaine wrote. But then one day Joanne told her that the doctors had said that there were no more drugs for Richard. They did ask permission to try one more medication just to see if it elicited any response. When Elaine tried to console Joanne by suggesting that it might turn out to be the miracle drug they were all waiting for, she made no response, and Richard died the following day.[31]

There also would be no miracle for Scott. A few years after Richard's death, a doctor gave Elaine and her husband the same terrible news Joanne had received—their son no longer could benefit from treatment. But the doctor recently had returned from Seattle, where researchers were conducting pioneering work on bone marrow transplants. If the parents agreed, Scott would be the first patient with Hodgkin's disease to receive that type of graft. "I was deeply thankful that there were still possible cures for Scott, that we had not exhausted every resource," Elaine remembered. "I kept thinking of what Joanne had told me about Richard. 'There are no more drugs they can use,' she had said sadly. But there was this new procedure for Scott. Perhaps this would be it. I was excited and hopeful." Excitement and hope were short-lived, however. Scott never was well enough to undergo the procedure.[32]

Gerda Lerner's memoir of her husband's illness and death is the rare account published in the 1970s expressing reservations about the motives of medical researchers, though she, too, honored their enterprise. Her personal history helps to explain her initial skepticism. As a refugee from Nazi Austria, she undoubtedly knew of the horrendous abuse of research subjects in concentration camps. Moreover, she had long been a political activist. After arriving in the United States, she joined the Congress of American Women, a communist-affiliated group, and organized poor African American women. Later she participated in trade unionism, the civil rights movement, feminism, and the movements against both McCarthyism and the Vietnam War. We can assume she closely followed the achievements of the women's health movement, which led the campaign to challenge male physicians' power.

But, as we have seen, she was an academic as well as an activist. Perhaps as a result, she respected the monopoly of knowledge that other professionals claimed. "In dealing with a complex disease like a brain tumor," she wrote in 1972 after Carl's diagnosis, "one is in an area where it is difficult for the layman to make judgments or evaluate the judgments of others. I understand only too well the pitfalls of operating outside of one's own limited field of competence. . . . My approach was to provide a team of experts, let them arrive at a collective judgment and insist that they interpret it honestly and openly to Carl and me."[33]

After Carl underwent surgery and radiation, his two primary doctors disagreed about whether he should submit to an experimental course of chemotherapy, and Gerda had no choice but to become involved. The surgeon, Dr. Ambrose, opposed further treatment, arguing that chemotherapy for brain tumors was still in the experimental stage and reliable statistics were not yet available. In addition, Ambrose, like Ellen Levit's Dr. Lorin, stressed the importance of easing the dying process. He noted that people dying from brain cancer experienced little pain and often were unaware of what was happening. Because chemotherapy weakened the immune system, Carl might well die from an acute infectious disease rather than from the brain tumor and thus experience greater suffering. The oncologist, Dr. Goldman, agreed that chemotherapy might produce dangerous side effects but pointed out that it offered Carl his only chance for a remission. Gerda initially sided with Dr. Ambrose, whom she had often described as wise and humane; she had especially been impressed by the unusual sensitivity he had displayed in his personal interactions with Carl. She also agreed with Ambrose's comments about the importance of considering the quality of Carl's last days. And she never had liked Goldman, considering him young and arrogant, with a brusque, occasionally contemptuous, manner.

Gerda also knew he was engaged in chemotherapy research. "There was no doubt in my mind as to his medical ethics or scientific integrity," she wrote, "but up to then I had seen little evidence that he considered his patients as individual human beings." She clearly did not misunderstand the purpose of clinical trials. "Might not [Goldman's] judgment be warped by overriding interest in the research?" she asked. "Once started, would Carl be able to have some control over his treatment or would he simply be a guinea pig in a scientific experiment? Such thoughts, admittedly, were neither fair nor charitable and I certainly had no grounds for my suspicions. Still, they were in my mind, and possibly they should be in the mind of anyone considering such a treatment."[34]

If Gerda questioned Goldman's motives, she had no doubts about the ultimate value of his work. Because the decision about chemotherapy rested with Carl, Goldman presented his arguments to him as well. "Someday," Goldman asserted, "we will find a way to cure brain tumor. I have absolutely no doubt of it. . . . Every patient who takes part in the research project, takes part in that search and contributes to it." Carl responded that although he liked that idea, his goal in pursuing chemotherapy was not to help others but to try anything that possibly could help his fight for survival.[35]

In her journal entry included in the memoir, Gerda recounted a very different conversation that occurred when Goldman tried to persuade Carl to continue the treatment even after both realized it probably was ineffective. As Goldman spoke about his mission, she "perceived something noble and grand in his passionate hatred of this enemy. . . . Somehow, the way he put it, there was some meaning in participating in that venture, that battle, which will go on when one's own life ceases. For a moment . . . he was on the same battleground with us, not because of us or of Carl as a person, but because we shared a common enemy. As an old political fighter, Carl sensed this and warmed to it. 'Okay,' he said and thanked [Goldman], patting him on the arm with a feeling of real warmth." In that version, Gerda not only asserted that medical research had a transcendent purpose but also presented Carl as wholeheartedly embracing it himself.[36]

AIDS

More than any other event, the AIDS epidemic that emerged in the early 1980s transformed the relationship between researchers and human subjects. Investigators had to deal not only with individual patients and their families but also with a highly motivated, well-informed, and politically experienced activist community demanding the right to participate in planning, conducting, and evaluating research studies. Less concerned than earlier critics about the pressures on patients to enter trials, people with AIDS and their advocates focused on barriers to access. "The nightmare image," historian David J. Rothman commented, "shifted from an unscrupulous researcher taking advantage of a helpless inmate to a dying patient desperate to join a drug trial and have a chance at life."[37]

Paul Monette's best-selling and critically acclaimed *Borrowed Time: An AIDS Memoir* enables us to feel the rage animating treatment activists. Monette and his partner Roger Horwitz, a lawyer, had lived in Los Angeles for ten years by 1985, when Horwitz was diagnosed with AIDS. That year the death toll from the epidemic had reached four thousand. Reading obituaries and watching opportunistic infections devastate the lives of friends. Monette knew Horwitz faced a dark future unless new and better treatments suddenly appeared. And then, two months later, Monette learned he himself was HIV-positive, thus adding a new level of urgency to his activism. The first sentence of his memoir read, "I don't know if I will live to finish this."[38]

Monette and Horwitz joined "a community of the stricken who would not lie down and die. All together, we beat down the doors of the system and made it take our count." As members of an underground medication distribution system, they traveled to Mexico to obtain ribavirin, an experimental antiviral drug produced by a small pharmaceutical company in southern California. Monette also breached the boundary between medical and lay knowledge. We saw that Gerda Lerner described herself as a reluctant student of her husband's condition. One of the hallmarks of AIDS activism, in contrast, was a determination to spread medical expertise to patients, their lovers, and their families. Monette claimed success in mastering the intricacies of medical science. "No explanation was too technical for me to follow, even if it took a string of phone calls to every connection I had," he asserted. "In school I'd never scored higher than a C in any science . . . but now that I was locked in the lab I became as obsessed with A's as a premed student. Day by day the hard knowledge and raw data evolved into a language of discourse."[39]

Although Monette and Horwitz belonged to a community of sufferers, they also enjoyed rare advantages. As Monette acknowledged, they had important connections and plenty of money. During his many hospitalizations, Horwitz stayed on UCLA Medical Center's exclusive 10-East, a wing with private rooms and concierge service. And one of his friends was willing to use his contacts in both government and academia to surmount "the high fence of experimental drug research." Within weeks of his diagnosis, Horwitz had received permission to enter the clinical trial of Surinam, one of the first drugs to hold out substantial promise as an antiviral agent. Later he became the first person west of the Mississippi to receive AZT, the "elixir" of the day.[40]

Two women's narratives highlighted the difficulties encountered by most people seeking medications in the 1980s. Four years after musician Keith Avedon died in 1987, his widow, Elizabeth Cox, published a narrative about his diagnosis and death. Toward the end of Avedon's life, a doctor had advised him to travel to Mexico for ribavirin, but customs officials were now more aggressive in confiscating the drug at the border. The weekly US cost of $100 was prohibitive to Avedon. Many other patients could not overcome rigid eligibility criteria that excluded them from trials. When Carol Lynn Pearson informed her four children that their father, her ex-husband, had AIDS, she assured them that "doctors and researchers are working night and day on finding a cure." And when Gerald told her he might be a candidate for the interferon trial scheduled to begin in a couple of months, she exulted, "I knew the researchers wouldn't let us down. . . . Any week now, any day now, they would announce the cure." But Gerald soon was diagnosed with tuberculosis, which barred him from the experimental treatment. Carol was aghast. "'But, but Doctor,'" she sputtered. "I couldn't let him go without some kind of hopeful statement—*anything!*"[41]

Patients who qualified for trials often endured long waits to enroll. Barbara Peabody was living in San Diego in the winter of 1984 when her ex-husband phoned to say that their son Peter, a struggling musician in New York, had AIDS-related pneumonia. She rushed across the country to visit him in the hospital and brought him back to her home as soon as he was able to travel. Seven months later, he received his first good news. DHPG, a new drug to treat cytomegalovirus (CMV), was about to be distributed on an experimental basis, and the doctor wanted Peter to enter the trial as soon as possible. But a week later Barbara learned that the pharmaceutical company would not release the drug until Peter underwent various medical evaluations. "I boil with anger and frustration," she wrote. "For God's sake, I want to scream. . . . My son may go blind and crazy without this one chance." When Peter received the requisite test on August 1, she complained about "the morality of the situation, that scientific method has priority over possible alleviation of suffering. I constantly hear talk about maintaining the 'quality of life' for the patient. And meanwhile, Peter is losing his vision, facing recurrent seizures and dementia, and his very life goes down the waste pipe in torrents of diarrhea."[42]

All the tests were complete by August 21, but Peter still had to wait for a bed to open in the research wing of the hospital. Barbara could not decide "whether to scream or cry. . . . I'm beginning to wonder if he will ever receive this drug, or will it simply be too late by the time they have all the rules and regulations fulfilled? I feel a desperate resignation. Maybe it doesn't even matter anymore. Maybe he's too far gone for help. He weighs

111 pounds tonight, six less than two weeks ago." Peter finally received the first dose of the experimental medication at the beginning of September. Two months later he was gone.[43]

Although AIDS activists focused primarily on the exclusionary practices of researchers and drug companies, access was not the only issue. In the absence of approved therapies in the early years of the epidemic, the line between experiment and treatment was extremely fluid. A doctor at New York Hospital later told an interviewer that he had "been involved in the experimental care of a number of [well-known AIDS patients], getting them drugs that no one had access to or trying things that didn't pan out, just to do something." But now informed consent forms enabled patients and families to learn about some of the dangers of treatment before it began. Elizabeth Cox's husband was one patient who read a consent form carefully. In her October 1986 diary entry, Cox noted that Avedon's doctor was trying to obtain AZT for him. Troubled by the list of possible complications he saw, Avedon showed her the release form. "Terrifying," she wrote. "I feel we are entering a twilight zone of not knowing which is worse, the illness or the cure. Such an awful frustration, not knowing what to do." Like many other people with AIDS, Avedon expressed his disappointment with mainstream medicine by trying alternative treatments, and he recently had received a supply of Tibetan drugs. "Western medicine, Eastern medicine," Cox mused, "What will happen if Keith takes them together? What will happen if he doesn't? What will happen?" Not surprisingly, she yearned for an established course to follow. By the time the AZT arrived, Avedon had developed CMV-induced retinitis and had begun to take DHPG, the drug Barbara Peabody's son had waited so long to try. Now the doctor was unsure how the two drugs would interact. "With the DHPG the risks of AZT are even greater than what the release form says, so it's hard to feel optimistic," Cox wrote. "We're both nervous."[44]

Novelist Fenton Johnson recalled that because his lover, Larry Rose, a high school teacher, could not tolerate AZT, the doctor switched him to ddI, a newer experimental drug. When Rose brought the first batch of ddI home, he had a sheaf of papers requiring both his signature and that of a witness. He read a grim litany of possible side effects, "up to and including death." Rose complied with the regime, but nonadherence was common. Mark Doty recorded such an incident. A major American poet, Doty had received numerous awards by the time he published *Heaven's Coast: A*

Memoir, an elegy to his lover Wally Roberts, who died of AIDS in 1994. Doty noted that for a while Roberts took ddl regularly, "even though we were full of questions: better to take an unknown drug or allow the body to do its own work? Which was more deadly, the invisible disease, the invisible treatment? . . . Neither of us really believed it was doing anything, but what might happen if he *stopped*?" But then Roberts had a bout of neuropathy, and he did end treatment. When the neuropathy receded, he began again, "but only half-heartedly. Soon it was hit and miss, an envelope here and there, nothing regular. Boxes of the little foil envelopes of medicine arrived by Federal Express, and we stashed them away in a kitchen cupboard; soon we'd have more and more of them."[45]

Unsurprisingly, some doubts subsequently received confirmation. Clinical psychologist Jean M. Baker, remembering the agony of watching her son Gary become sicker and sicker, wrote that the constant preoccupation of everyone with AIDS was "to decide between taking highly toxic medications with potentially dangerous side effects or leaving potentially lethal infections untreated." Every morning Gary injected his thigh with granulocyte-macrophage colony-stimulating factor (GMCSF), believed to increase white blood cell counts. "He was stoic and uncomplaining as he carried out his daily ritual," his mother wrote. "GMCSF was an experimental treatment, and Gary was among the first in the country to participate in the clinical trials. . . . It was only later that GMCSF was found to be ineffective and perhaps even dangerous as a treatment for AIDS-related problems."[46]

When UCLA discontinued its Surinam study, Monette wondered whether he had been too quick to demand that Horwitz receive the drug. "Nothing said Roger had to be on an experimental therapy within weeks of his hospitalization or else. Indeed, now I see how innocent we were about just how uncertain experiments can be." As the memoir closed, Monette was grateful that AZT had extended Horwitz's life for nine months but furious that the drug had not been available earlier. Present-day readers know that researchers soon announced that AZT also was too toxic and ineffective.[47]

Clinical Trials for Advanced Cancer after 1980

Although AIDS had the most dramatic effect on the medical research enterprise, the media continued to report examples of abuse in clinical trials for other diseases, especially cancer. In 1981 a series of articles in the *Washington Post* charged that the MD Anderson Cancer Center had treated patients like guinea pigs, administering drugs that were so toxic that several participants died. Moreover, the research was at a very early stage. Since the late 1960s, the Food and Drug Administration had required investigators to study drugs in three distinct phases. The MD Anderson study was a Phase I trial, which meant that the purpose was to investigate dosage and toxicity. It also meant that participants' chance of reaping any direct personal benefit was virtually nonexistent. Soon after those articles appeared, the US House Committee on Energy and Commerce, Subcommittee on Health and the Environment, held a hearing to investigate the accusations. Prominent physician researchers extolled their progress in conquering a deadly disease, emphasized the urgent need for more studies, and lambasted the regulations that curtailed their work. Defending the use of highly toxic drugs in clinical trials, Dr. Vincent DeVita, director of the National Cancer Institute, declared that "the most serious toxicity of all is the unnecessary death from cancer." Emil J. Freireich, a professor of medicine at the University of Texas System Cancer Center, pronounced the new regulatory regime "toxic to patients who currently have cancer" and "toxic to those of us who will in the future develop cancer." Edward N. Brandt, assistant secretary for health, Public Health Service, stated that patients who had exhausted all known treatments "welcome any chance for benefit, no matter how slim."[48]

Throughout the postwar period, large numbers of doctors had insisted that patients on the verge of death were eager to participate in experiments. Brandt, however, spoke at a very different time. Testifying at the same hearing, Alexander Capron, executive director of the President's Commission for the Study of Ethical Problems in Medicine and Biomedical and Behavioral Research, contended that doctors should offer patients no longer likely to be cured not only another experimental treatment but also supportive services, including pain relief. As we will see in chapter 6, the hospice movement began in 1974; by 1981, hundreds of programs were either in existence or being planned. Espousing a new model of end-of-life care, hospices provided an alternative to the endless pursuit of innovative interventions. In addition, patients in the early 1980s were far less willing than those in previous decades to defer to the judgment of doctors and researchers. Following the lead of AIDS activists, advocates for people with cancer demanded and slowly won participation in decisions that set the research agenda. And individual patients and relatives acted more assertively, searching on their own for experimental regimes, rejecting some trials their doctors recommended, and refusing to adhere to protocols that seemed to serve research interests alone.[49]

Jean Craig, the head of a Los Angeles advertising agency, already had lived through a husband's terminal illness when she met Ed McNeilly, another advertising executive. Soon after they married and moved to a large house in Malibu in 1986, a doctor informed McNeilly he had metastasized colon cancer. McNeilly had no doubt that he could find physicians and clinical trials on his own. His first step was to fire his doctor, who had tried to dissuade him from getting another opinion. The second was to learn all he could about experimental programs. "We'd decided to go beyond conventional treatment," Craig explained. "Maybe there was something going on experimentally that would give us a shot." Telephoning the National Cancer Institute, McNeilly heard about the Physician's Data Query (PDQ), which listed all clinical trials in the United States, and requested a copy. Craig described what next happened: "Ed found twenty-nine institutions on the PDQ printout doing programs directed against colon cancer. 'I'm going to talk to them all, Jean. And I'm going to do it myself. I don't trust anyone to do this for me.' He picked up the telephone. And began calling them, one by one." After interviewing various researchers in the Los Angeles area, McNeilly entered an experimental protocol at the City of Hope.[50]

Others refused to enroll in recommended trials. John A. Robertson, a professor at the University of Texas School of Law and a national expert on medical ethics, wrote that his wife's doctor suggested that she join a study rather than receive the standard treatment for her type of cancer. She declined because the study would have involved travel to a distant cancer center. She preferred to stay home and continue teaching as long as possible. Will Schwalbe's mother, Mary Anne, understood that the Phase I trial to which she was referred was unlikely to extend or improve her life. Perhaps because she had devoted much of her life to public service, she felt she had a moral obligation to participate. In this instance, however, altruism was not enough. The trial would have involved additional hospitalizations, tests, and invasive procedures. Choosing to focus on the quality of life rather than its quantity, she enrolled in a hospice.[51]

Sidney Winawer explained why he gradually supported his wife's desire to deviate from a research protocol. Andrea Winawer was in the midst of an experimental trial for stomach cancer at the University of Wisconsin when her psychiatrist suggested she also receive interferon. Sidney, a prominent physician and medical researcher at the Sloan-Kettering Cancer Center, had many objections. He knew that the small doses of interferon recommended for Andrea would have little chance of success. They might, however, interfere with her other treatment; almost certainly, they would inflict further suffering. Above all, because Andrea knew her oncologist would not allow her to take both treatments simultaneously, she intended to travel to Atlanta to receive the medication without informing him. "Trial protocols are inviolable," Sidney wrote. "Only with the careful data records they provide can conclusions about their effectiveness be made and guidelines for treatment drawn." As a husband, however, he now understood what AIDS patients and their advocates had long asserted: "The dying have no time for research. . . . When a life is at stake, the life of someone you love, you want to pull out all the stops. Throw every weapon you can get your hands on at a disease, and in the end, if the patient lives, who cares what worked and what didn't." After reading reports of various studies, he decided to violate the "sacred rules" of his profession and accompany Andrea to Atlanta.[52]

Many more patients bypassed their physicians' authority by obtaining advice from the World Wide Web. After his son's melanoma returned, Richard Lischer discovered that the Internet made it "possible to shop for treatments the way one searches for the best hotel buys or the cheapest airline tickets. It is not difficult to hook up with a hospital representative online, to indicate one's preference for a specific doctor or treatment, to jet down, say, to Houston, and to be streamed into the assessment system of a major cancer center, all inside a week's time." One guide advised patients to take control of their care: "Understanding current availability of clinical trials requires time and due diligence, something many physicians lack. You must search out the appropriate trials available for your specific tumor-type, always advocating in your own best interest towards a cure." According to David Rieff, his mother, Susan Sontag, adopted such an aggressive approach. Soon after learning she had myelodysplastic syndrome (MDS), an extremely lethal variant of blood cancer, she was on the Internet feverishly searching for any treatment that might show even a hint of promise.[53]

But the use of the Internet could have a downside. Although none of the memoir authors mentioned any suspicions of the medical websites they consulted, some may not have contained accurate information. Some websites also may have encouraged inflated expectations about what clinical studies could deliver. As bioethicist Rebecca Dresser writes, "In presenting clinical trials as cutting-edge treatment," those sites "reinforce patients' belief that research is equivalent to treatment." Moreover, unlike Paul Monette, some people eventually acknowledged the limits to how much medical information they could acquire and the treatment decisions they could make on their own. "Even my mother," Rieff wrote, "so supremely confident in her own ability to 'work up' subjects and master information, found herself incapable of following what she was being told." He added, "[I] felt much the same way, as if I had suddenly found that I had become a functional illiterate. There was all this information, but it was in a foreign language." Although John A. Robertson's wife ultimately refused to enroll in a study, he began looking on the Internet for ovarian cancer trials as soon as he learned the diagnosis. He found many ovarian cancer trials discussed online, but none seemed to be appropriate for his wife's condition. "And, without medical expertise," he acknowledged, "I couldn't tell whether my impression was correct."[54]

Amanda Bennett had a similar realization. Bennett worked for the *Wall Street Journal* in 2000, when her husband, Terrence B. Foley, a linguist and a musician, was told he had a rare form of kidney cancer. Using the skills she had honed as a journalist, Bennett immediately began "obsessively prowling" the Internet. "There were tantalizing signs that something was changing in cancer treatment," she wrote. Foley underwent therapy, but the cancer returned eighteen months later. By that time the number of research programs had burgeoned. As a result, Bennett was able to show the oncologist "a fistful of printouts. Names of Doctors. Names of hospitals. Names of drugs and descriptions of clinical trials." But she finally acknowledged that she could not evaluate the studies she had found. Her research did, however, lead her to Dr. Ronald M. Bukowski, a kidney cancer expert at the Cleveland Clinic, who recommended that they do nothing while waiting to see how the disease continued to develop. Placing their faith in Bukowski, Bennett and Foley accepted his advice. "For all our research," Bennett wrote," it wasn't really the science we were following. It was the people. We took the measure of the people we trusted and then followed the path they led us on."[55]

Trust in an individual practitioner, however, was not a precondition for investing enormous hopes in an experimental regime. Although Meghan O'Rourke's mother knew that enrolling in a study represented a "last ditch effort," she was shocked to learn that the therapy had not prevented the spread of tumors to her brain. Meghan informed the research oncologist of this latest development. Later, she recorded their conversation:

> "*Real*-ly," he said slowly. His response was dramatic. But his tone was not the one I had hoped for. He didn't sound embarrassed or apologetic. Instead, he sounded *intrigued*. "That's highly unusual," he drawled.
>
> Then, gathering himself, he said, "I'm sorry to be so clinical about it. I know this is your mother, but that is fascinating. This rarely happens with colorectal cancer." . . .
>
> "Yes," I said, stunned into monosyllables by his assumption that I could think clinically about the fact that renegade cells were devouring my mother from the inside out.

Meghan was even more aghast when the doctor proceeded to stress how much he had learned from patients like Barbara, her mother. But because he did not say that the setback would mean the end of the mother's experimental therapy, Meghan retained a glimmer of hope. Only when an administrator phoned the next day to say that Barbara would be discontinued did Meghan acknowledge that her mother really was dying.[56]

Two patients enrolled in recommended trials after learning that their doctors previously had concealed critical knowledge. Richard Lischer recalled that his son Adam had laughed bitterly when his doctor told him that although his relapse was extremely serious, he could enter a clinical trial. "It was a quickie, heard-this-one-before laugh," Richard wrote, "because only sixteen months earlier we *had* heard this before—about a clinical trial with interferon." Adam had entered a clinical trial earlier, after his initial diagnosis. At the time, no doctor had informed him that a previous study had found that although melanoma patients treated with interferon had longer remissions, they did not live any longer. Nevertheless, Adam participated in the new trial he was offered. The other patient was Terrence Foley. Despite the determination of Amanda Bennett and

Foley to adhere closely to Dr. Bukowski's instructions, their trust in him faltered at one point. When Foley's tumor showed signs of growth, Bukowski urged him to join a clinical trial. Like many AIDS patients and their families, Foley and Bennett were horrified to read the severity of the side effects listed in the consent form. They also discovered two other issues Bukowski had failed to disclose. One was that he was an investigator and thus had an interest in encouraging eligible patients to participate. The second was that it was a Phase I trial and unlikely to benefit Foley. He did, however, enroll in the next trial Bukowski recommended. (Much later he and Bennett learned that Bukowski was a researcher on that trial as well.)[57]

Even as the end approached, some patients and family members refused to relinquish the hope that a new intervention might reverse the outcome. When Foley lay near death in an intensive care unit, Bennett urged the resident to continue treatment while they waited for the latest investigational drug to work. And David Rieff wrote that Susan Sontag "subscribed with her whole being to a deep assumption regarding contemporary medical research—at least as it exists in the public mind—which is that cures will eventually be found for most if not all diseases." That faith had sustained her during two previous bouts of cancer. When she again became ill, she "hoped to be able to find solace and strength in it once more, even though realistically, with MDS, and at her age, the bad odds of surviving any advanced cancer had become prohibitive." She flew across the country to undergo a bone marrow transplant that caused harrowing problems and had only a remote chance of success. Returning to New York after that procedure failed, she embarked on an experimental drug that inflicted further suffering. As a result, Rieff concluded, "Hers was the opposite of an easy death."[58]

Conclusion

The patients and family members described in the memoirs were exceptional in two respects. As individuals with relatively high social status, they probably were especially likely to resist medical authority. It is thus notable that even they frequently regarded their doctors as saviors. In addition, because I chose only memoirs in which the patient died after a long illness, the accounts may have been especially bleak. Some experimental treatments are effective, and some patients prevail. Had I selected some of those treatments and patients, I might have presented at least a few cases with positive outcomes.

The stories recounted in this chapter occurred against the background of a decline in medical dominance. The recurrent exposés of abuse of human subjects, the demand that physicians disclose diagnoses, the growing emphasis on informed consent, and the expansion of popular medical knowledge helped to shift the balance of power from doctors to both patients and their families. In the early 1980s, patients and family members began to adopt a more assertive stance vis-à-vis medical researchers. Rather than scrupulously following doctors' orders, they searched on their own for information about clinical trials, decided which ones, if any, served their interests, and disregarded accepted protocols. Nevertheless, the growing autonomy of patients and families can easily be exaggerated. Evidence suggests that some of the websites lay people view as repositories of unbiased information misrepresent clinical studies, exaggerating their benefits for participants and downplaying the risks. Even highly educated individuals have found the information on the Internet so abstruse and overwhelming that they have turned to one physician as the arbiter. And a refusal to defer to medical experts has not always led to a more realistic appraisal of experimental treatments. Some people have continued to believe that the next study, against all odds, could produce miraculous results.

The psychology of illness may help to explain why people often overestimate the therapeutic value of clinical trials. "One does not despair if one can act, and if one can hope that the action will be rational," wrote social theorist Zygmunt Bauman. "One can keep despair in abeyance as long as one *acts:* as long as one knows that not all has been lost, that 'something can be done yet.' . . . Rational efforts go on draining the abysmal depths of irrationality. They will never reach the bottom, but at least one need never again think of the bottom unless the effort stops." Since the end of World War II, clinical studies have helped to divert thoughts of mortality. As long as there was one more novel therapy to try, patients and their loved ones could ignore the overwhelming likelihood that the story would not end happily. The following chapter explores how individuals responded when inflated expectations met a harsh reality.[59]

3

When Medicine Fails

The search for clinical trials at the end of life might seem to represent the triumph of the view that biological factors alone explain physical disease. Medical successes buttress that assumption. Antibiotics cure many bacterial infections; insulin keeps diabetes under control; surgery removes malignant tumors; experimental treatments sometimes extend lives. But the writers of many of the memoirs examined in this book wanted medicine to do more. As we saw in chapter 1, some felt betrayed by doctors who refused to acknowledge the depth of their anguish or address existential issues. And all eventually had to admit that some illnesses could not be fixed.

Beyond Conventional Treatment

Historian Anne Harrington argues that when mainstream medicine disappoints "by failing to validate fully the complexity of one's suffering" or "by being unable to deliver a cure," people begin to search for narratives about how the mind affects the body. The titles of two books popularizing what we now call mind-body medicine appeared over and over in the family memoirs. In *Anatomy of an Illness as Perceived by the Patient*, Norman Cousins recounted his own experience of recovering from a disease with a terrible prognosis by watching humorous films and television shows and reading comic literature. Bernie Siegel's *Love, Medicine, and Miracles* sought to show that patients who harnessed their inner resources had the power to heal themselves.[1]

Although Harrington argues that mind-body practices gained force partly from their deep roots in religion, she ignores what religion itself offers people confronting serious illness and death. The memoirs suggest, though, that religion has a much larger place in the lives of very sick patients and their families than any form of mind-body medicine. Most of the people in those accounts who sought mind-body healing indicated that, like a majority of Americans, they believed in God. Indeed, far more memoirs discussed reliance on religious resources than on any type of mind-body medicine. This section first examines people who pursued mind-body healing and then turns to those who looked to religion either to promote recovery or to infuse the experience of illness and death with meaning.

Harrington claims that "the stories of mind-body medicine are at their most powerful when they . . . inspir[e] people to turn their backs on conventional remedies, defer to new kinds of healers, embark on unaccustomed travels, [and] undertake new kinds of practices." Several memoir writers, however, viewed mind-body healing as intimately connected to participation in clinical trials. Sidney Winawer's wife Andrea, we recall, underwent an experimental treatment for stomach cancer, which she supplemented with interferon. But she never placed her faith in medical care alone. Returning home one evening, Sidney was startled to find Andrea reading a book by Bernie Siegel. He admitted that, "like many conventional doctors," he previously had viewed Siegel with suspicion. But as he watched Andrea gain strength from Siegel's writings, Sidney changed his mind: "Patients facing lethal diseases have to find hope, and the start of hope is the belief that they can help themselves. Help themselves to survive, if that is possible. At the very least, help themselves to live well and die by their own rules, not those of the disease." Andrea's insistence on making her own treatment decisions thus won his praise. She was becoming "the kind of patient Bernie Siegel writes about. She was energized, empowered, bent on knowing the options and then choosing her own way."[2]

Jean Craig attributed even greater significance to the self-determination that Sidney Winawer gradually learned to appreciate. Cousins's *Anatomy of an Illness* had been her "touchstone" from the beginning of her husband Ed McNeilly's struggle with cancer. Later she also found inspiration in Bernie Siegel's writings. Thus, when McNeilly announced he had decided to enroll in a City of Hope trial after interviewing a large number of researchers, she exulted that "in only a little more than a few weeks he'd taken control of his situation" and added, "With control comes strength." He had changed "from a man terminally ill who was going to be kept comfortable, to a man fighting, in charge, living—and, the most amazing thing of all, to a man who was happy." Toward the end of McNeilly's life, Craig returned to that theme. As she watched him laugh at a movie about an "indomitable American soldier" in the Vietnam War, she realized McNeilly was the same type of man. Throughout his long illness, he had drawn on "the reservoir of strength" that was part of the American character. "We're optimists," wrote Craig. "We like to crack jokes in the face of danger. We're taught from birth to admire 'rugged individualism.' We're taught from birth to believe any one of us can accomplish whatever we put our minds to. 'Yes. You can grow up to be President,' our children are told. And they can." McNeilly's impending death might have demonstrated how little control he exercised over his destiny. Instead, Craig cast him as the exemplar of the self-sufficient American man, able to triumph over all adversity.[3]

The belief in mind-body healing had special appeal to the many people with HIV/AIDS who believed, often with good reason, that mainstream medicine had abandoned them. Barbara Peabody's son Peter was gravely ill with AIDS in May 1984 when he learned that his friend Jack had died from the same disease. Peter was sad but not unduly concerned about his own future, because he believed Jack had had the wrong attitude. "[Peter] wants to believe that a positive attitude will conquer all," his mother wrote. "Indeed, sometimes his faith is so strong, I find myself believing he will succeed." The long delay in his entering an experimental protocol thus terrified her not only because increasingly dangerous symptoms continued to besiege him but also because she worried he would lose heart. "Greater than my fear of losing him," she wrote, "is the fear of the day when he realizes there will be no miracles and he will have to surrender hope." Each new postponement seemed to hasten that event.[4]

Several writers asserted that they and the patients believed in the possibility of miraculous healing, not only from a medical breakthrough or mind-body practices but also from some form of divine intervention. Researchers conclude that people's level of belief in divine intervention varies inversely with their socioeconomic status, as defined by income and education. Had this book focused on families and patients with lower status, we might expect to find a very high proportion believing that events unfold according to a divine plan. It is thus especially significant that large numbers of memoir writers demonstrated at least some faith in miraculous healing.[5]

Ann Hood's memoir began, "The day my father was diagnosed with inoperable lung cancer, I decided to go and find him a miracle." A novelist and short story writer, Hood understood that "for some people the notion of seeking a miracle cure is tomfoolery, futile, or even a sign of pathetic desperation." But the family already had sought various medical options, and none had offered hope. As a result, she traveled to Chimayo, a town in the Sangre de Cristo Mountains in New Mexico, known as the "Lourdes of America." There she entered the church, scooped up some reddish soil believed to have healing powers, and said a prayer. She then carried the dirt in a Ziploc bag back to her father in Rhode Island. The day after he received the dirt, a doctor reported that the tumor had disappeared. Nevertheless, Hood's father soon died.[6]

Although Hood no longer believed a medical cure was possible when she went to Chimayo, other writers placed their faith in religion and scientific medicine simultaneously. After assuring her children that doctors were working hard to cure their father's disease, Carol Pearson commented, "And we'll do our part too. We'll continue our prayers." Soon after Mary Winfrey Trautmann's daughter Carol began cancer treatment at Los Angeles's City of Hope, a local minister reminded Trautmann that she could serve as the channel through which the Holy Spirit flowed. As a result, she began reading about miracles and healing and attending meetings at a charismatic church. There she found "an attitude and an atmosphere that sustain hope and promote courage."[7]

A few writers described special healing ceremonies. Terry Tempest Williams recalled participating in a Mormon service for her mother on the eve of her surgery for ovarian cancer. "At dusk, we moved inside to the living room and created a family circle. Mother sat on a chair in the center." The eldest son "anointed Mother with consecrated olive oil to seal the blessing." Next, men who belonged to the highest priesthood "gathered around her, placing their hands on the crown of her head. My father prayed in a low, humble voice, asking that she might be the receptacle of her family's love, that she might know of her influence in our lives and be blessed with strength and courage and peace of mind." Kneeling next to her grandmother, Williams "felt her strength and the generational history of belief Mormon ritual holds. We can heal ourselves, I thought, and we can heal each other."[8]

Le Anne Schreiber was another daughter who participated in a healing ritual in her mother's behalf. Schreiber had just moved to the Hudson River Valley when her mother was diagnosed with pancreatic cancer. During the following eleven months, Schreiber traveled frequently to her mother's home in Minnesota to deliver care. Although Schreiber no longer subscribed to any religious affiliation, her mother was Catholic. When the mother told her priest that she was about to have cancer surgery, he invited her to a special Mass of Anointing. After the priest placed a drop of oil on her forehead and each palm, the other worshippers began to file by. Then, in Le Anne's words,

> Each person stopped, placed both hands on Mom's head, blessed her and wished her well. Every one of them was a true believer in the healing power of God, and the intensity of concentration they brought to their moments of contact with Mom was overwhelming. With few exceptions, they looked straight into her eyes, expressing an unaccountable intimacy and a deep desire to pass on something healing in their touch. . . . As they continued to file by, Mom gripped the top of the pew with both hands, looking as if she were holding on against a strong, steady wind.

Schreiber continued that her mother "clearly felt that powerful medicine was being administered, and so did I. I had never felt such intensity of good will, and if nothing more than that were at work in this chapel, it was enough to quiet my skepticism." It would be impossible to disentangle the social dimension of the ceremonies from the religious element in these two events. We can speculate that both mothers may have gained sustenance from the communities surrounding them as well as from the spiritual rituals enacted.[9]

Although Schreiber may have been at least somewhat more willing to believe in the power of prayer after witnessing that ceremony than before, faith in divine healing often coexisted with doubt. Madeleine L'Engle was a writer best known for her young adult fiction; her most famous book, *A Wrinkle in Time*, won the 1962 Newbery Medal. "What about prayer?" she asked in 1988 after recounting the grueling cancer treatment her husband Herb, an actor, had endured. Despite the "literally hundreds" of prayers that had been said on his behalf, the news was unremittingly bad. And yet she found some solace in her faith. She was unwilling to believe those prayers were "wasted" or "lost." "I do not know where they have gone," she wrote, "but I believe that God holds them, hand outstretched to receive them like precious pearls."[10]

Doubts also assailed Gordon Livingston, a psychiatrist who believed in both mind-body healing and religion in addition to mainstream medicine. A month after his six-year-old son Lucas was diagnosed with leukemia, Livingston wrote that he was steeped in "the literature of hope," including works by Bernie Siegel and Norman Cousins. Livingston thought "all the time about what more we can do to support [Lucas's] spirit and perhaps thereby increase the probability of healing. We're hoping to do so by creating an environment so filled with determination that he inhales it with the air he breathes." As the word "perhaps" indicates, Livingston was far from convinced that what he called "attitudinal healing" would be effective. Nevertheless, when Lucas was able to return to school after his first round of chemotherapy, the father credited not only the treatment but also Lucas's emotional resilience and cheerfulness.[11]

Livingston had begun to question the existence of God long before Lucas was diagnosed with leukemia, and he thus approached prayer the way he did attitudinal healing—hoping against hope that evidence of efficacy would overcome his skepticism. After learning that Lucas would need repeated hospitalizations and chemotherapy, Livingston wrote that he found comfort in the "firmly religious people we have heard from who are asking God's help in ways in which they truly believe. I hope that their certain faith redeems my poor agnosticism when the Almighty weighs the fate of my poor son." But when Livingston himself prayed, he feared it would be clear that he did so only under duress: "My prayers, such as they are, reek with the fraudulence of a battlefield conversion." Because two cycles of chemotherapy failed to halt the disease, the oncologist suggested a bone marrow transplant. Ten days after the procedure began, a cold kept Livingston from the hospital. "I went to church by myself," he wrote, "and prayed with a sincerity I can recall only from my youth when last I truly believed."[12]

Patients and family members used religious resources in other ways as well. If a belief in God could not prevent death, the notion of an afterlife might soften the blow. When Terry Pringle realized that his four-year-old son was losing his battle with leukemia, Terry envisaged himself sitting by the boy's bed and explaining what he believed about death: as Eric's spirit left his body, "he will find that he is above us, able to look down on this mourning family. He will no longer be in pain and will be overcome gradually with the great peace that he has been released from the sufferings of the world, a world that he can now see but from which he has been separated. Then he will move off and return to God." Pringle did not indicate to what extent he actually believed in the possibility of life after death and to what extent he was trying to convince himself that his beloved child still could have some form of existence.[13]

Finally, spiritual resources helped people prepare for mortality. As a theologian, Richard Lischer must have been exquisitely attuned to the spiritual path his son Adam followed. Departing from his father's faith, Adam began receiving instruction in Catholicism soon after meeting his future wife, Jenny. When he learned that his melanoma had spread to his brain, Adam quit his job as a lawyer and intensified his religious devotion. "We are going to use our time in a new way," he told Jenny. Together, they "lit candles, said their prayers, recited the psalms, went to daily Mass, did the Stations, [and] knelt at icons." Adam had long been interested in the Bible, but now his Bible reading had what his father called a "vocational focus," to determine how he and his wife should understand his impending death. By reflecting his suffering, the psalms helped to fill a void in the health care system. "Medical science is deaf to suffering," Richard explained. "It responds to pain when it can be connected to a physical problem and quantified. 'On a scale of one to ten, how would you rate your pain?' But suffering, with its many depths and its mysterious interplay of body and spirit, is beyond the scope of pain and therefore beyond the competence of most medical practitioners. There were times when Adam wanted to tell somebody about his sadness, fear, or anger, but the hospital provided no acoustic space for that kind of talk." When a terrible headache descended shortly before his death, Adam asked Jenny to read from the psalms to him. He "closed his eyes and tried to absorb the ancient medicine directly through the outer membrane of his forehead and into his swollen brain."[14]

Whereas Adam underwent extensive therapy while devoting much of his energy to religion, other narratives described relatives who rejected further treatment as they prepared for the end. Barbara Rosenblum, a sociologist, found solace in the Judaism of her background. She and Sandra Butler, a feminist writer and activist, had been partners for six years when Rosenblum was diagnosed with advanced breast cancer at age forty-two. After several rounds of chemotherapy failed to halt the disease, she refused a bone marrow transplant, the one remaining therapy. As Butler wrote, "The risks of losing quality time because of the side effects" of that treatment "were too great to balance the statistically equivocal benefits." Rosenblum's final months represented a "sacred time." Meeting regularly with a rabbi to prepare for death, she gradually realized she was part of a larger whole. A few weeks before Rosenblum died, Butler noted that the

Jewish teachings "give her comfort now, a sense of place and of time, and ability to see herself on a continuum between life and death, between the past and the future, between her beloved grandmother, dead now for decades, and her two-year-old nephew."[15]

We saw that Terry Tempest Williams's mother Diane drew on her Mormon faith during her struggle with ovarian cancer. When Diane learned that a friend had just been diagnosed with a brain tumor, she sent a letter describing her experience twelve years earlier while undergoing an operation for breast cancer:

> During the surgery, I had a spiritual experience that changed my life. Just before I awakened in the recovery room, I was literally in the arms of my Heavenly Father. I could feel His love for me and how sorry He was that He couldn't keep this from me. What He could and did give me was far greater than not having cancer. He gave me the gifts of faith, hope, strength, love, and a joy and peace I had never felt before. These gifts were my miracle. I know it is not the trials we are given but how we react to these trials that matters.

A sense of intimacy with the natural world as well as Mormonism helped Diane adhere to those lessons when she confronted a new set of trials. Terry noted that the family believed "that God can be found wherever you are, especially outside. Family worship was not just relegated to Sunday in a chapel." As Diane endured two operations, two rounds of chemotherapy, and several weeks of radiation, she found renewal in the deserts, mountains, and gorges surrounding her Salt Lake City home. After rejecting yet one more kind of chemotherapy, she began the process of dying. Echoing Sandra Butler, Terry characterized that final period as "a sacred time."[16]

Sociologist Robert Wuthnow argues that American religion increasingly has moved toward a "spirituality of seeking." Sara M. Evans, a professor of history at the University of Minnesota, used similar terminology, characterizing her mother Maxilla as "a spiritual seeker who discovered her affinity for Quakerism after a lifetime as a Methodist minister's wife." After she refused both a final round of chemotherapy and invasive procedures for her heart, she lived in what Sara described as "a grace-filled limbo." Maxilla, too, approached nature with reverence, and it provided her with a constant source of fascination and joy. A year before Maxilla died, Sara wrote that her mother "is still my teacher when it comes to living peacefully with uncertainty." Even as her health steadily declined, Maxilla continued to delight in her flowers and tomato plants. "That connection with the world of living things is an amazing source of sustenance to her," Sara commented.[17]

Many memoirs, of course, made no mention of religion. Others discussed it only to highlight its absurdity and irrelevance. Roni Rabin was in college when her father, a professor of endocrinology at Vanderbilt University, received a diagnosis of amyotrophic lateral sclerosis (ALS). Roni acknowledged that religious beliefs might have eased the family's painful experience during her father's five-year struggle with the disease. But Roni's psychiatrist mother "was a critical thinker who looked at everything closely, holding each issue to the light, turning it to all sides the way she'd examine a dress for stains before buying it. 'Who can believe in God after World War II?' she'd ask. And that was that. The bottom line. That one sentence of hers set the tone for religion in our house." The father's illness "merely confirmed the atheistic tendencies all of us shared. No God would let such a cruel and horrible thing happen. Period."[18]

Marcia Friedman became incensed when a friend tried to convince her that her son's premature death represented the mysterious working of God's will: "If I had believed in God before Josh got sick," Friedman wrote, "I sure as hell wouldn't now. Why Josh? Because he's always been good? Bright? Handsome? What kind of irrational 'pattern' or 'plan' would that be? I was furious." According to David Rieff, Susan Sontag was irate when a Buddhist friend sent a note assuring Sontag she was inside a Buddhist circle of protection and would definitely recover. "This is *grotesque*," she said, throwing the letter on a table.[19]

Even some people who viewed illness and death through a religious framework were alienated by church positions on social issues. Bobbie Stasey repeatedly emphasized the sustenance she received from her intimate relationship with God when she cared for her son with AIDS. But driving to the hospital one day, she passed a church with a sign in front. Expecting to find an inspirational message, she was horrified to read, "AIDS IS GOD'S PUNISHMENT TO HOMOSEXUALS." Her memoir continued: "I couldn't believe what I was reading! 'NO!' I screamed, pounding my fist on the steering wheel. 'How dare they say God is punishing my son! They have no right!' . . . I shook uncontrollably. 'He doesn't deserve that. No one deserves that! Fuck that church and everyone in it! I hope they burn in hell!' "[20]

Le Anne Schreiber had not expected to be moved by a healing ceremony, because she had previously left the church as a result of its positions on women's issues. Nevertheless, the day after the ceremony, she entered another chapel and began to pray for her mother. Although loath to relinquish her anger about the church's stance on social issues, she "allowed that maybe the church knew something I didn't about sickness and death, maybe it was better at comforting the dying than guiding the living." But then, on the way out, Schreiber stopped to peruse the pamphlets on a table. "I picked up one titled, 'Mamma, Why Did You Kill Us?' and began to read. It is the allegedly factual account of a last confession given by a woman who has been visited by all the unborn fetuses she had aborted. I put fifty cents in the donations box and took the pamphlet with me so that I could rekindle my anger in the place of my choice."[21]

But if some memoirs were filled with antireligious comments, others testified to what religion could offer people confronting terminal illness. Some memoir writers looked to divine intervention for the miraculous cures medicine had failed to provide. For some, the notion of an afterlife alleviated the pain of loss. And many relied on spiritual resources to frame the experiences of suffering that medical science could not prevent.

Acceptance

The inability of medicine ultimately to avert death not only has encouraged reliance on both mind-body healing and religion but also has helped to elevate the cultural value of acceptance. That development both counters the emphasis on intensive, high-tech therapies at the end of life and provides a new script many dying individuals are expected to follow.

Although resignation to God's will was a key element in the nineteenth-century concept of a good death, the current, more secular version of acceptance owes much to the influence of Elisabeth Kübler-Ross's 1969 book *On Death and Dying*. The core of her argument was that mortality had become taboo in American society. Unable to face their own anxieties about death, doctors prolonged life after virtually all hope of recovery had ended and failed to communicate honestly with the dying. Families and friends, she argued, dissimulated their feelings or withdrew, thus heightening patients' sense of isolation. And denial kept everyone from understanding what was really important. "It is from our dying patients that we learn the true values of life," she wrote in a later book, "and if we could reach the stage of acceptance in our young age, we would live a much more meaning-ful life, appreciate the small things, and have different values."[22]

Kübler-Ross's example of a good death was that of a farmer she had known as a child in Switzerland, a country that had just begun to rely on medical technology. After falling from a tree, the farmer realized he could not survive. His only request was to die at home. Once there, he "called his daughters into the bedroom and spoke with each one of them alone for a few minutes. He arranged his affairs quietly, though he was in great pain, and distributed his belongings and his land. . . . He also asked each of his children to share in the work, duties, and tasks that he had carried on until the time of the accident. He asked his friends to visit him once more, to bid good-bye to them." Having made those preparations, the farmer was ready to die.[23]

Kübler-Ross also accorded an honored place to acceptance in her fa-mous theory of the grief process. Based on observations of dying hospital patients, she concluded that people close to death passed through five emotional stages: denial, anger, bargaining, depression, and finally accep-tance, the zenith. Patients who arrived at the last stage, she asserted, ap-proached death with serenity. Family members moved through the same stages either before or after the death occurred.[24]

Working closely with hospital chaplains, Kübler-Ross emphasized the role of religion in helping people achieve acceptance. One of her examples of a patient who successfully reached that state was a very religious man who spoke frequently about the solace he received from his intimate con-nection to God. His wife found strength in the Bible and believed that her husband's fate was in God's hands. Kübler-Ross later asserted that people who genuinely believed tended to move through the same emotional stages as others but did so more quickly and with less difficulty. She also insisted, however, that faith was not a prerequisite. Any patient who "is allowed to grieve," whose "life is not artificially prolonged," and whose "family has learned to 'let go' . . . will be able to die with peace and in a state of accep-tance." In her 1997 memoir, Kübler-Ross recalled, "My dying patients never healed in the physical sense, but they all got better emotionally and spiri-tually. In fact, they felt a lot better than most healthy people." The benefits extended to family members. Those whose dying relatives had attained acceptance could find the final hours enriching rather than depressing. Kübler-Ross's model has been widely challenged. Critics contend that she idealized the dying process, prescribed rather than described dying patients' psychological responses, and vastly underestimated the power and pervasiveness of denial. Nevertheless, the theory remains highly influential.[25]

In the years since Kübler-Ross wrote, both the use of aggressive treatments near the end of life and opposition to them have increased. By 2009 nearly 30 percent of people age sixty-five and over who died spent time in an intensive care unit (ICU) in their last months of life. Commentators explain that figure in various ways. The culture of medicine encourages patients, family members, and doctors to assume that death can be endlessly postponed and that more treatment is always better. In addition, some patients believe they have a responsibility to act heroically, submitting even to the most painful procedures. Because many doctors provide either no prognoses or overly optimistic ones, patients often are unaware they have little chance of survival. Family members fear they will feel guilty if they do not press for the most aggressive treatments. Equating death with failure, physicians refuse to admit defeat.[26]

Financial incentives also encourage doctors to offer more and more therapy. Until July 2015, Medicare paid for the administration of procedures but not for talking with patients about living wills and advance directives. The first attempt to change those incentives ended in failure. During the 2009 debate about federal health care reform, one proposal was to reimburse physicians for holding voluntary conversations with patients about their end-of-life wishes. But Sarah Palin denounced those conversations as "death panels," a charge that right-wing politicians and talk-show hosts endorsed and repeated. Senator Chuck Grassley, of Iowa, argued that Americans had "every right to fear" that the provision would require "pulling the plug on Grandma." Two independent polls found that 30 percent of the population agreed that conversations about advance planning represented death panels. In deference to public opinion, the Obama administration soon dropped the proposed regulation. (It was reinstated six years later, after the furor had died down.)[27]

If some people feared that so-called death panels might limit their chance of survival, however, many others express terror at the prospect of dying tethered to machines, alone in an ICU. Thus, the movement to humanize care of the dying has steadily gained force. That movement receives support from various studies indicating that many dying people receive far more aggressive therapy than they want. According to researchers at the Dartmouth Institute for Health Policy and Clinical Practice, the amount of treatment patients receive is most closely correlated with the supply of health care services in the area rather than with patient wants or needs. Other studies have found that the major concerns of people close to death are to alleviate suffering, remain in control of their lives, prepare for death, help others, achieve a sense of completeness, and receive affirmation, not to prolong life. Still other studies have reported that most doctors are unaware of their patients' end-of-life preferences and that although nearly three-fourths of people state they want to die at home, just one-third actually do so. The high cost of end-of-life treatments has intensified opposition to them. One frequently cited figure is that one-third of Medicare funds go to people with chronic diseases in the last two years of life.[28]

To many champions of more humane ways of caring for dying people, acceptance of mortality is the essential first step. After recounting several stories to illustrate problems with the American way of dying, journalist Stephen P. Kiernan concluded, "The real challenges are attitudinal—that people who are dying accept their condition, that loved ones join in that recognition, and especially that society organize itself around the idea that death with dignity is appropriate and attainable." Writer Katy Butler's 2013 *Knocking at Heaven's Door* was basically a diatribe against the new technologies that "seemed to have blunted medical staff to the suffering their procedures caused the dying, and often postponed death without restoring health." For several years she had tried to persuade doctors to deactivate her father's pacemaker as his mental and physical health steadily deteriorated and caregiving increasingly consumed her mother's life. Despite Butler's failure to have the pacemaker turned off, her father finally entered a hospice unit, where he died peacefully. Butler entitled the section describing that death "Acceptance." In Atul Gawande's widely acclaimed 2014 book *Being Mortal,* he noted the importance of "arriving at an acceptance of one's mortality and a clear understanding of the limits and possibilities of medicine." And Abigail Zuger, another physician, reviewing that book, praised Gawande for defecting from the "army of doctors bent on preserving life" to the "tiny band able to accept death."[29]

While Elisabeth Kübler-Ross looked to the Switzerland of her youth for the model of an individual who died well, more recent commentators often turn to the nineteenth century, when popular culture urged dying people to show fortitude in the face of pain and suffering, accept God's will, and provide evidence of salvation. Despite the danger of conflating prescription and description, some commentators suggest that most people acted in accordance with those ideals. More recent examples of good deaths also provide instruction. "How to Die" was the title of a 2012 account in the *New York Times* of a death in the United Kingdom, where strict protocols prevented futile interventions. "Unfettered by tubes and unpestered by hovering medics . . . he died gently, loved and knowing it, dignified and ready." By contrast, Jonathan Rauch's 2013 *Atlantic* article "How Not to Die" included several instances of people who received unnecessary and unwanted treatment that inflicted suffering at the end of life.[30]

Three individuals who appeared to have faced death with equanimity and integrity have received especially widespread acclaim. Soon after Cardinal Joseph Bernardin died in November 1996, his photograph appeared on the cover of *Newsweek*. The accompanying article, entitled "The Art of Dying Well," began, "For the journey everyone must face, Cardinal Joseph Bernardin illuminated the trail." Three months earlier Bernardin had written a public letter announcing that his pancreatic cancer had returned and that, although he had less than a year to live, he was at peace. "As a man of faith," he wrote, "I see death as a friend, as the transition from earthly life to life eternal." According to *Newsweek*, he used his final months to complete a book, make arrangements for his ninety-two-year-old mother, try to heal divisions in the church, and "reconcile himself to God."[31]

The following year, Mitch Albom's *Tuesdays with Morrie* offered a nonreligious account of the pursuit of acceptance. A newspaper sports writer, Albom recounted his weekly conversations with his former sociology professor, Morrie Schwartz, who was dying of amyotrophic lateral sclerosis (ALS). Displaying no self-pity, Schwartz expressed gratitude for having had a life filled with meaning, being able to say goodbye, and learning to cherish every minute. He urged Albom to reorient his priorities, living as if he really knew he would die. Albom's book was a bestseller, has been translated into thirty-one languages, and was adapted as both a play and a television movie.[32]

Randy Pausch's death in 2007 seemed especially poignant because he was relatively young (forty-seven), in the midst of a thriving career as a Carnegie Mellon professor, and the father of three children under age six. Pausch had just agreed to deliver a prestigious annual lecture at his university on computer science when he learned that his pancreatic cancer was back and he had three to six months to live. Changing the title of his presentation to "Really Fulfilling Your Childhood Dreams," he spoke about his illness, his determination to live the rest of his life as fully as possible, and his hopes for those who survived him. The talk was captured on video and soon went viral on *YouTube*. During the following months, he appeared on the *Oprah Winfrey Show*, ABC News named him one of its three "Persons of the Year" for 2007, and *Time* included him in its list of the world's one hundred most influential people.[33]

Pausch became even more famous after his death with the publication of *The Last Lecture*, cowritten with a *Wall Street Journal* columnist. He distilled the lessons he had learned from his life and enjoined his readers to treat others well, set high goals, and never give up. He also made it abundantly clear that he had no illusions about his future. He expressed his wishes for his children as they grew older and explained what he wanted them to know about him. He noted that he had moved the family to a different state, where they would have relatives to help after his death. And he emphasized his thankfulness that he and his wife had been able to "work to come to terms with what her life would be like" when he was gone. That book, too, became a bestseller, and it has been translated into thirty languages.[34]

Most of the family memoirs used in this study similarly assigned a high value to acceptance of death's inevitability. Having had to face the fatal illness of beloved kin, writers were acutely aware of prevailing attitudes. "Dying is un-American," wrote Doris Lund. Journalist Andrew H. Malcolm concurred: "In most families, death is the *d*-word, not to be spoken. One day Grandma . . . speaks over Sunday dinner. 'Someday when I'm gone—,' she says. But her voice is drowned out by her offspring and their spouses," who assure her she will live forever. The children "get the message that death is right up there with sex on the list of family unmentionables." Malcolm found the source of American attitudes in the isolation of dying people in hospitals and the adoption of new technologies to prolong life. Other writers focused on the triumphalism following World War II, when the country emerged as a seemingly invincible power. "Those of us born after the war were raised in an era of mass forgetfulness," Le Anne Schreiber wrote. "Death was put behind us."[35]

Many memoirs also explained how the cultural denial of death compounded the difficulties of caring for and ultimately losing loved ones. As we saw in chapter 1, some authors charged that physicians who could not acknowledge the reality of death failed to disclose bad news. Some writers also complained about the evasions of other health professionals. Alan Shapiro remembered his disbelief in the enforced cheerfulness of the physical therapist he encountered in his sister's hospital room shortly before her death. Joyce Guimond, a nurse herself, recalled that when her eight-year-old son was dying in an intensive care unit, the nurses cared for him with skill and compassion. But they "seemed committed to a cheerful assumption that all would be well, in spite of the fact that we knew he was dying." The conversations in the room were "always general, almost social in nature, and no one seemed able to talk with us about what was uppermost in our minds. Namely, how could we bear this tragedy? How could we and his brother and sisters attempt any sort of normal living again?" Guimond concluded her article with advice for her colleagues: "Attempts on the part of nurses to show empathy, to understand, and to communicate more understandingly with families who suffer the death of a child would not only help them in accepting and coping with their immediate anguish, but would probably make the long adjustment easier to endure."[36]

The flight of friends heightened relatives' sense of loneliness and isolation. The first person Doris Lund told about Eric's leukemia "flinched as if I struck her." "People hardly want to hear such news," Lund continued. "Their eyes tend to slide away." Even a former college roommate who had been a friend for twenty years begged Lund not to tell her more than she could stand. When Janet Bode was dying, her partner Stan Mack turned to friends and neighbors for assistance, "with mixed results. Some simply could not face Janet's illness."[37]

In addition, the narrative writers praised patients who had reconciled themselves to the end. We saw that some memoirists described relatives who had relied on spiritual resources. Others told of people who achieved some level of acceptance in the absence of faith. Ann Hulbert was the literary editor of *Slate* and the author of two well-received nonfiction books when she wrote "To Accept What Cannot Be Helped," which appeared in the *American Scholar* in 2010. Her article stressed the benefits of acceptance but made no mention of any form of religion. Hulbert's eighty-year-old mother had a long history of resisting medical interventions of all kinds. When she learned she had inoperable brain cancer, she decided not to submit to chemotherapy and radiation despite the doctor's contention that they might ease her symptoms and add a few months to her life. "She wanted to escape the dingy hospital corridors," Hulbert explained, "the endless waits, the nurses who dragged their feet and addressed her and my father as though they were dim children, the doctors who urged procedures knowing she was a patient with top-notch health insurance." Instead, she spent the summer in her house in the Berkshires, surrounded by her large family. Religion also was absent from Mary Jumbelic's story about her mother's death. As a medical examiner, Jumbelic was very familiar with death as a natural part of life when her mother was diagnosed with metastatic pancreatic cancer. She, too, declined chemotherapy and radiation. "We went on a family cruise," Jumbelic wrote, "my husband, our kids, mom, and I. We savored the time together; we rested, relaxed, and prepared emotionally for what lay ahead." Neither mother had the peaceful death Kübler-Ross promised. Hulbert's mother hallucinated on the morphine she needed to keep the pain under control. Jumbelic's "heart nearly broke" when she moved her mother's body on her final day and saw that "the slightest turn caused her excruciating pain." Nevertheless, both mothers found an alternative to the endless pursuit of medical treatment.[38]

But several memoirists discovered that acceptance was not what everyone wanted or needed. A common complaint today is that the emphasis on natural childbirth has created a set of rigid expectations for birthing women and that some women feel like failures when they cannot conform. Similarly, several writers charged that the current focus on acceptance has imposed a new model on dying patients that is not always appropriate. Kathryn Temple, a professor of English at Georgetown University, described her husband's response to the news that he had a rare, extremely lethal cancer. "From the day of diagnosis," Temple wrote, "he rejected his six-to-twenty-four-month prognosis. He fired doctors who insisted on discussing it, replacing them with those more willing to speak positively about 'treatment' and 'options.'" Although he grew weaker, his heart failed, and he was rejected by every transplant hospital in the area, he refused to believe he might not get better. In an advance directive before major surgery, he indicated that he wanted every form of intervention to keep him alive, including feeding tubes and respirators. "No measures were to be rejected in pursuit of life." When hospital administrators demanded that Temple remove her husband to a hospice, she tried to discuss that option with him. With the help of a remote, he turned the television volume high enough to drown out her words.[39]

Temple initially hewed closely to the ethic of acceptance: "I felt strongly that my husband needed to understand his prognosis, that understanding would allow him to make choices about his treatment and his legacy, bring him closer to his family and friends, and, in short, help him face his future in the full knowledge of what his life had meant and would mean." As she learned about the function of denial as a coping mechanism, however, she changed her mind: "I began to believe that he should be respected for the choice he was making, that he was choosing to believe in a future that made him feel whole. It was not my right to impose my own negative, 'realistic' view on that choice."[40]

Joseph Sacco also could not force a family member into the acceptance script. When he graduated from medical school in the early 1980s, he had received no instruction in death and dying except for a single video describing Elisabeth Kübler-Ross's theory of grief. Thus, when his father was diagnosed with incurable cancer a few years later, Sacco assumed that his primary mission was to act as a guide through her five stages. His father occasionally asked for the truth but refused to hear it, and despite his rapid deterioration, he remained convinced he would beat his illness. "Once so intent on enforcing my own version of a good death, a death of acceptance," Sacco wrote, he gradually realized that he had to accompany his father "on the path of his own choosing."[41]

Le Anne Schreiber similarly discovered that the acceptance paradigm did not meet a parent's needs. When her mother's health sharply worsened a month before she died, Le Anne's brother repeatedly urged her to help their mother reach the stage of acceptance. Each time Le Anne tried to broach the subject of death, however, her mother diverted the conversation. "None of us want Mom to end her life in confusion or depression," Le Anne commented after several abortive attempts, "but do any of us have the right to strip her of hope?" Until recently their mother had had good reason to assume she would recover. The doctors had encouraged her in that belief, and Le Anne assumed her mother's optimistic attitude had enabled her to withstand a horrendous therapy. "Suddenly she is being confronted by defeat, and it is not easy to adjust, not easy to abandon the stance that has allowed her to endure as long as she has." When her sister-in-law phoned to ask if the mother had accepted the fact that she was dying, Schreiber wrote, "It is easy for someone at a distance to think there is some abstract state called 'acceptance of death' and that you can maneuver a sick person into it at your convenience. Here, on location, Mom is not cooperating."[42]

A few authors of memoirs suggested that denial had benefits for themselves, not only the patients. Some wanted to escape the dominion of illness. With her deep belief in the power of positive thinking, Jean Craig was proud that her husband Ed McNeilly never allowed metastatic colon cancer to derail his life. When her first husband had been terminally ill, the family was not "tainted by illness. It was normal." She again "fought hard for normalcy" after McNeilly learned he had metastatic colon cancer. "The best thing you can do when you're ill," she declared, "is to live as if you're not." Two weeks after major surgery, when McNeilly was still receiving pain medicine and trying to adjust to his colostomy, he planned a trip to London. When a doctor told him his tumor was growing and warned him not to make any major investments or buy any new businesses, he purchased a car wash. Unlike the many patients and family members who complained about friends who disappeared, McNeilly and Craig refused to let others share their suffering. When they held a joint birthday party six months after McNeilly's diagnosis, Craig avoided looking at the one couple who knew he was sick. "I didn't want cancer in the room," she explained. "I wanted my birthday with Ed and I was glad—so very, very glad—that people were sharing the moment with us as if it were just a silly party for a couple of silly friends. Had they all known, we couldn't have thrown the party. Too maudlin. Too touching. Too many smiles forced onto worried faces. Instead it was normal and filled with laughter." Several months later, Craig's advertising agency held its annual beach party near their house. Although McNeilly had just had an infusion pump installed, he "dropped in for an hour or so, his pump hidden in his windbreaker, his Heparin lock under his shirt, his chemical dripping into his arm, and laughed and joked and ate barbecued chicken as if he hadn't a care in the world."[43]

John A. Robertson finally agreed with his wife that they should confine illness to the margins of their lives. His wife went through major surgery and many rounds of chemotherapy after her diagnosis with stage four ovarian cancer. During that time he repeatedly tried to talk with her about death, but she invariably refused. "She realized that talking and sharing would have made it more difficult for both of us," he wrote after her death. "And she was right. Neither one of us wanted the cancer to be center stage, with the klieg lights of fear and panic shining in the darkness. We wished the cancer would fade away and disappear, but knew that it wouldn't. So, we had to deny and distance."[44]

Unlike the many writers who extolled the virtues of either acceptance or denial, Mark Doty found uses for both. A poet, he illustrated what John Keats called "negative capability," the ability of the great artist to embrace openness and live with ambiguity and uncertainty. After his partner Wally Roberts was diagnosed with AIDS, a woman asked Doty how he felt about knowing he would lose his lover. Doty responded that he *"didn't* know." Anything could happen. Doty could die first, a cure might suddenly appear, or Roberts might survive for a long time with his disease. "It seemed important to me to maintain that kind of openness," Doty explained, "to resist fatalism." But he also acknowledged that he saw a "slow erasure of Wally taking place." "In my heart," Doty wrote, "I felt this process as inexorable. We were moving downward, on the charred slopes, and nothing I could do would stop it."[45]

Later, Doty attempted to summarize his stance. He and Roberts "tried to steer a course between fatalism and an unacceptable optimism." Like Jean Craig, the two men desperately wanted "normalcy." Somehow they had to continue to engage with the world "in the light of new and extraordinary knowledge." But they also were aware that any sense of normalcy they achieved was "founded in part on denial, on forgetting." When Roberts still was able to go to work each day, Doty wrote, "we'd go on as if we were fine and then crash and go on again."[46]

One anthropologist notes that "abstractly considered, the idea of caring for someone dying at home focuses primarily on the idea of death." In practice, however, "caring for the dying is very much about life and helping the dying person to live out what is left of life. In most cases the fact of death remain[s] in the background, crowded out by the intense demands of caregiving." In his discussion of Roberts's final weeks, Doty made a similar point. Now it would have been impossible to pretend that anything resembling normalcy existed. Roberts spent his days in a hospital bed, was incontinent, could barely communicate, and had little understanding of events around him. Doty had full knowledge of what lay ahead, but like Le

Anne Schreiber, he did not argue that acceptance must be everyone's goal. In his case, pressure to produce the proper emotions came from a professional rather than a family member. Visiting the house for the first time, a nurse asked Doty whether he had made funeral arrangements. When he resisted her attempts to engage him in discussion, she decided he was experiencing denial. Her arrogance enraged him. "I'm not in denial," he wrote. "I'm just hanging on trying to get through the day." Doty was even more aghast when the nurse interpreted Roberts's brain dysfunction as denial and decided that he, too, needed counseling. Although Doty forbade her to talk with Roberts, she proceeded to ask him whether there was anything he still wanted to do that he had not yet done. "At this point," Doty wrote, "you might as well ask my lover a question in Swahili."[47]

Conclusion

"It has become a bit too trendy to regard the acceptance of death as something tantamount to intrinsic dignity," wrote the paleontologist Stephen Jay Gould, recounting his successful battle with an especially lethal form of cancer. Gould's comment overestimates the extent to which acceptance has become a fashionable value. We have seen that many patients and family members view a fight to the finish as the best way to preserve dignity and that a very high proportion of doctors pursue cure at any cost. And a key concern of many memoirists was to counter the widespread denial surrounding them. Even if they shared relatives' fight to retain normalcy, they wrote about serious illness and death and thus exposed life's essential fragility and medicine's ultimate limitations. But several writers also echoed Gould's complaint about the pressure on dying patients to come to terms with their own mortality. A few memoirists discovered that at least some degree of denial was necessary to continue to enjoy what was left of life. Others had tried unsuccessfully to guide their dying relatives toward acceptance before concluding that all individuals must find their own way to approach finitude. If emphasis on the acceptance of mortality serves as a welcome antidote to the growing emphasis on aggressive and often futile treatments at the end of life, it also imposes a rigid model on the emotional responses of gravely ill people and their families.[48]

4

Caring by Kin

Preventing Stress and Preserving Dignity

In the early 1980s, researchers and policymakers suddenly discovered family caregiving. One reason was a dramatic demographic shift combined with women's increased participation in the labor force. The elderly, who constituted 4 percent of the population in 1910, had increased to 11 percent by 1980. Although most people sixty-five and over can care for themselves, approximately one-quarter require at least occasional help, and the prevalence of disability rises steeply with age. As the proportion of women with waged work increased from 44 percent in 1960 to 67 percent in 1990, policy analysts and government officials increasingly worried about who would be available to care for the growing elderly population.[1]

Reports about escalating Medicaid costs heightened that concern. A joint federal-state program originally intended to assist poor women and children, Medicaid directed 44 percent of its funds to nursing homes in 1983. That year the Reagan administration sought to save money by encouraging states to reduce access to Medicaid facilities, thus shifting caregiving responsibilities back to the home. Medicare expenditures for acute care also came under scrutiny. Changes in the way Medicare reimbursed hospitals for patient care resulted in a drop in the length of stay. One researcher estimated that five years later hospitals had transferred 21 million days of care work to homes. It was thus crucial that family members, especially women, be up to the job.[2]

Alzheimer's Disease

Perhaps more than any other factor, a new understanding of Alzheimer's disease helps to explain the growing visibility of family caregiving. No longer conceptualized as senility, age-related cognitive decline was redefined as a specific disease with distinctive symptoms and pathological processes. A recent college graduate, Marion Roach had just begun a job at the *New York Times* in 1979, when she learned her mother had Alzheimer's disease. Roach later recalled that she and her sister "looked everywhere for more information, for help. We became pack rats of ideas. There was no listing in the telephone book, no entry in the encyclopedia. We already knew what the dictionary said about senility. It said nothing about Alzheimer's disease." But that year saw the establishment of the Alzheimer's Disease and Related Disorders Association (the ADRDA, later the Alzheimer's Disease Association), dedicated to increasing public awareness of the condition. In a series of widely publicized congressional hearings in the early 1980s, association leaders emphasized the prevalence of Alzheimer's disease and the problems it posed for families as well as patients. Unlike people with most other serious chronic diseases, those with dementia primarily require supervision and help with routine daily activities, not medical services. Family members rather than doctors and nurses thus provide the great bulk of the care.[3]

ADRDA also helped to launch a caregiving research industry. According to PubMed, the federal government's database for journal articles in medicine and the life sciences, the annual number of articles on caregiving jumped from 3 in 1980 to 857 in 2015. By the end of 2015, a total of 7,520 articles on the subject had been published. Recent studies demonstrate that families are the core of the long-term care system. Although estimates of the number of caregivers vary, a 2009 survey reported that 48.9 million people had provided care to an adult relative during the past twelve months. Two-thirds of the caregivers were women. The average number of hours per week devoted to caregiving was 20.4. The cost of replacing those services was a staggering $450 billion.[4]

The Institute of Medicine reported in 2008 that fear of a dwindling supply of caregivers had led to repeated "calls to increase the support that is provided to them." Those calls have largely gone unanswered. The Medical and Family Leave Act, passed to widespread acclaim in 1993, covers leaves of no more than twelve weeks, provides for no remuneration, excludes part-time and contingent workers and those employed in small firms, and defines families very narrowly. Workers who are white, middle-class, and married have been the ones most likely to take advantage of the act. Many state programs have similar restrictions; those that provide paid leaves typically exclude elder care. The national Family Caregiver Support Program, established by Congress in 2000, is directed toward caregivers with low incomes. States receive money to inform clients about available ser-

vices and facilitate access and to provide counseling, support groups, training, and respite care. The program's funding level is too low to enable states
to furnish substantial assistance.[5]

While policies to provide substantial help to caregivers have lan-
guished, the self-help industry, including workshops, books, articles, au-
dio and video products, and personal coaching, has flourished. Most are
directed to family members of people with dementia. The first manual for
that group appeared in 1981, soon after the reconceptualization of Alzheimer's Disease and the establishment of ADRDA. *The 36-Hour Day: A
Family Guide to Caring for Persons with Alzheimer's Disease, Related Dementing
Illnesses, and Memory Loss in Later Life,* by Nancy L. Mace and Peter V.
Rabins, contained a wealth of information about dementia, the major problems family members face, and the types of assistance available. Now in its
fifth edition, the book continues to be widely sold. And it has been joined
by a steady stream of other resources for caregivers.[6]

Stress reduction is the central theme of the advice directed to caregivers of relatives with dementia. The first step, they learn, is to recognize the
warning signs, including anger, irritability, loneliness, and exhaustion.
The second is to learn how to manage stress. Frustration and anger diminish when family members learn more about dementia and realize that many
of the most irritating behaviors are disease symptoms. Caregivers who employ tips for handling common problems can forestall major crises. Caregivers also must engage in various forms of self-care. And caregivers should
seek additional help from other family members and friends, community
services, and, eventually, institutions. Support groups are especially important because they relieve stress not only by countering isolation but also
by providing an opportunity for members to express unpleasant feelings
rather than keeping them under tight control. Finally, and perhaps most
importantly, caregivers should cultivate positive attitudes. "Instead of
dwelling on what you can't do," the AARP website advises, "pat yourself on
the back for how much you are doing and focus on the rewards of caring
for someone you love."[7]

The responses of the memoir authors to self-help advice varied. Twenty-
three of the narratives used in this book discussed care for relatives with
dementia. Most of the ones who published their works after 2000 described
themselves as enthusiastic consumers of the advice industry. Barry R. Petersen, a CBS News correspondent, was "forever reading books or checking

the latest website on Alzheimer's" to learn how to respond to the changes he observed in his wife Jan, another journalist. According to those sites, her deterioration would proceed inexorably through a series of predetermined stages, damaging and then ultimately destroying her sense of self. Quoting frequently from the "Seven Stages of Alzheimer's Disease," on the Alzheimer's Association website, he presented Jan's story as a case study.[8]

Petersen also learned how to monitor his own responses. In the summer of 2007, two years after Jan's diagnosis, he "realized how the personal toll on me was building. I was now the living embodiment of the new Alzheimer's book title: *The 36-Hour Day*." Recording his life the following spring, he quoted first from the "Ten Signs of Caregiver Stress by the Alzheimer's Association" and then from a newspaper article entitled, "Chronic Stress Can Steal Years from Caregivers' Lifetimes." When his weight and blood pressure rose precipitously, he knew he had joined the "legion of stressed out people where one in ten caregivers say their own health is worse."[9]

Although few other caregivers adhered so closely to the advice literature, many indicated that they read books and blogs, attended workshops and lectures, joined support groups, and consulted social workers and therapists. They, too, noted the importance of dealing with their anger and frustration. Knowledge about the genesis of irritating behaviors helped them gain control over those emotions. John Daniel's memoir *Looking After* described the four difficult years he and his wife spent caring for his mother, Zilla, after moving her from Maine to Oregon, close to their home. Zilla had been a labor organizer and now defined herself as a spiritual seeker. Daniel, a poet and essayist, was struggling with a mid-life crisis. Before he understood that his mother had Alzheimer's disease, he thought she had simply chosen to be evasive. Instead of responding to his questions about her life, she would comment only about irrelevant matters. Those remarks "recurred with maddening frequency." His anger dissipated when he learned that her mother's actions were unintentional.[10]

Knowledge about the typical course of dementia also helped to lower caregivers' expectations of what they could accomplish. Sue Miller was already a best-selling novelist in 1988 when she assumed responsibility for the care of her father, a former clergyman and academic. By learning about his condition, she was able to forgive herself for failing to halt his decline. "I think this is the hardest lesson about Alzheimer's disease for a caregiver:

you can never do enough to make a difference in the course of disease. . . . The disease is inexorable, cruel. It scoffs at everything."[11]

Nevertheless, several narratives harshly criticized the self-improvement industry. Two pointed to the lack of attention paid to economic issues. A short story writer and novelist chose to write his memoir under a pseudonym, Aaron Alterra, to protect the privacy of his wife of sixty years after her memory began to fail. "Considering the large role financing the illness plays in the life of most people with Alzheimer's," he wrote, "the literature has remarkably little to say about it. Excepting perfunctory suggestions to consult my lawyer or financial adviser, how the condition was to be paid for was excluded from every book about Alzheimer's I picked up." Like John Daniel, Eleanor Cooney had moved a mother across the country to be able to provide care, in this case from Connecticut to northern California. "The sages—advice books, help hotlines and such—presume a certain level of solid middle-class fiscal security and take it from there," Cooney wrote. Both she and her partner Mitch were freelance writers with unstable incomes, and caregiving consumed much of the time they expected to devote to work. Cooney quickly discovered that "without the protection of money, the strain starts to kill you right away."[12]

Two caregivers who were able to pay for much of the help they needed complained about the family values that undergirded some advice they received. *The New Old Age*, a *New York Times* blog, offended Alex Witchel, a staff writer for the *New York Times Magazine*. Witchel charged that many comments seemed to imply that she could be a good daughter only if she quit her job, neglected her marriage, and cared for her mother around the clock at home without assistance. Judith Levine criticized the prevailing assumption that family relationships invariably were filled with warmth and compassion. Best known for her controversial 2002 book *Harmful to Minors: The Perils of Protecting Children from Sex*, Levine has written about a wide variety of subjects, including aging, gender, consumerism, and popular culture. "Like most things about aging and illness in America," she commented, "the idiom of Alzheimer's has love written into it." Her arrogant, irascible father, with whom she had struggled throughout her life, had suddenly become "the loved one." Her major complaint, however, focused not on the content of the advice but rather on the use her mother made of it. The reigning caregiver narrative, Judith asserted, had encouraged her mother to exaggerate her burdens to justify divesting herself of responsibility. Judith had little sympathy for her mother's complaints about loneliness and lack of assistance. She challenged her mother's assertion that she had devoted the past ten years exclusively to caregiving and expressed disbelief when her mother insisted that all affection for her husband had vanished. When the mother announced she had been dating "Sid," whom she met in her support group, and she wanted to place her husband in a nursing home, Judith became enraged: "I'm determined not to let Mom represent herself as the victim of circumstances as scripted by the official Alzheimer's story. . . . The implication of such powerlessness is that the consequences of decisions—to be with Sid, for instance—are not really her own."[13]

Because Marion Deutsche Cohen, a poet and mathematician, cared for a middle-aged husband with advanced multiple sclerosis rather than an elderly relative with dementia, her diatribe does not, strictly speaking, belong in this section. Nevertheless, her criticisms might well resonate with many family members tending people with various conditions. Cohen's husband Jeffrey was a University of Pennsylvania physics professor when he was diagnosed in 1977 at age thirty-six. Cohen agreed that the next ten years, when Jeffrey still could care for himself, "might be described as [a period] of stress." During the subsequent six years, which ended with his entry to a nursing home, however, she was "in full-blown dire straits." Ordinary stress was something people might agree to do again, such as begin a new job, get married, or have a baby; by contrast, "dire straits . . . are not something a wise person chooses to repeat." "Well spouses don't suffer from ordinary stress," she declared. "We do not need stress-management workshops. . . . Calling dire straits stress undermines well spouses and makes us feel alienated and confused about where we stand." The major difficulties she faced stemmed from the inadequacies of the long-term care system and thus were not amenable to personal change. The mother of four children, she had total responsibility for a bedridden man who could not turn over, woke several times at night, and summoned her frequently during the day. Doctors, social workers, physical and occupational therapists, and other family members provided only minimal assistance. Eventually she found a service that furnished several hours of free attendant care each weekday, but she needed much more. She put the question she urgently wanted answered in the words of her son: "When's the government gonna decide we've had enough and do something about it?"[14]

AIDS

Emerging during the early 1980s, just when Alzheimer's disease garnered new attention and the movement of patients out of hospitals began, the AIDS epidemic created unique caregiving challenges. As a result, it, too, demands special attention. Before the advent of protease inhibitors and new antiretroviral treatments in the mid-1990s, the disease was almost invariably fatal. People with AIDS (or PWAs, as they were dubbed) often experienced a cascade of serious medical problems, including severe diarrhea, difficulty breathing, muscular skeletal pain, neuropathy, blindness, cognitive impairment, and dementia. The number of new diagnoses grew rapidly from 318 in 1981 to 75,457 in 1992. The death toll was 50,628 in 1995 alone.[15]

AIDS initially was known as the "gay disease" because gay men accounted for the great majority of early cases. Most were white, well-educated, and affluent. As the incidence of the disease increased, the composition of the affected population changed. By 1990 nearly a quarter of the cases were found among intravenous drug users. The overwhelming majority were poor, many were African American or Latino, and a significant number were women.[16]

The sixteen family memoirs I read about care for people with AIDS focused exclusively on gay men. As one scholar reminds us, narratives about that population "tend intrinsically to be the *best*-case scenarios." They typically "underplay, if not ignore completely, issues of money, insurance, transportation, housing, and transacting the business of paying bills and filing forms. This dichotomy between the typical case and those represented in print is perhaps truer of AIDS narratives than those of many other diseases, for two of the most heavily afflicted groups—gay men and intravenous drug users—tend to have different demographic profiles."[17]

"Families of choice" were the first line of defense for many gay men. Researchers report that between 30 and 40 percent of gay men were in committed relationships. When AIDS struck one member of a partnership, the other typically became the primary caregiver. Partners' accounts revealed the anguish of witnessing the devastation the disease wrought not only on loved ones but also on entire communities. Fenton Johnson, for example, saw his world drop away "person by person." After noting that one friend was likely to die soon, Johnson wrote that "his death would signal the end of an era of my life. Those first years of coming to San

Francisco, the first years, really, of coming out, of making peace with being gay—gladiolas and opera, discos and drugs, those will have wound to an end, and hardly in the way anyone might have expected. Of my old circle all would be dead except me." To Bernard Cooper, "keeping track of one's losses" became a "constant, morbid chore." He "tried not to extrapolate from every tragedy," but "certain deaths were especially foreboding" and he could not help making the connection to his lover.[18]

Unlike many of the caregivers of relatives with dementia, most gay partners of men with AIDS were relatively young. At a time when many of their contemporaries were building relationships and work lives, both people with AIDS and their caregivers were dealing with mortality. "Over and over," Paul Monette wrote, "I've watched those who are stricken fight their way back to some measure of health and go on working. . . . Perhaps the work is especially important because AIDS is striking so many of us just as we're hitting our stride." Listening to his seventy-five-year-old mother talk about attending the funeral "of one old friend after another," Fenton Johnson realized he had prematurely aged. "*Yes, I know this place,*" he thought, "*In my thirties, this is where I am.*"[19]

Partners also lacked many of the privileges of married couples. Some hospitals refused to allow partners to make treatment decisions and enjoy the same extended visiting hours as spouses. Beverly Barbo explained why she had to make funeral arrangements for her son. His lover "could not do this because a relative had to sign the papers."[20]

In addition, partners had to confront their own mortality. Men who had been tested at the same time as their lovers had an especially keen understanding of the arbitrariness of fate. Mark Doty recalled the morning a public health worker came to the house: "She told us our results. Me first, then Wally. I remember going and standing behind him. . . . I don't remember if he was crying, but I remember the stunned aura around him, the sense of an enormous rupture—not a surprise, but nonetheless a horror, an announcement fundamentally inadmissible, unacceptable. Shattering, but not a surprise, for had we been thinking of anything else? And though she must have told me my status first in order to deliver good news, before the blow, I remember thinking it didn't matter which of us it was, that his news was mine."[21]

Bernard Cooper "let out a long, pent-up breath" when a clinic counselor told him he had tested negative. But then he realized Brian had been in the consultation room for a long time. "I must have said 'Oh no' out loud, because a couple of people in the waiting room glanced in my direction. My muscles tightened, jaw clenched, body braced against the blow I feared most. Brian finally opened the door and signaled me inside."[22]

The sense of vulnerability never entirely vanished. As his lover's disease progressed, Doty found that people were "forever sizing me up to try to guess if I have AIDS or not—checking out my weight, whether my cheeks look hollow, or not, how tired I look." Cooper underwent testing a second time. During the hour before getting the results, he "paced in circles, checking the clock again and again. Fear leaked into my fingers, my feet. By the time I dialed the telephone, my thoughts were hazy and disconnected." Cooper's status remained unchanged, but some caregivers received their own grim diagnoses. After Paul Monette discovered he was HIV positive, he worried about what would happen when he developed symptoms: "There were so many stories now of desperately sick men being cared for by lovers who were just a hair's breadth behind."[23]

Families of choice also included friends and community members. Now editor-in-chief of the *Women's Review of Books,* Amy Hoffman was a member of a group of lesbians and gay men who banded together to care for Mike Riegle, a prison rights activist, in 1992. They cleaned his apartment, took him grocery shopping, raised money to pay for his medications, and visited him in the hospital. As his designated health care proxy, Hoffman made end-of-life decisions after he became incapacitated.[24]

A common assumption is that gay men received little care from people related by marriage or other traditional family ties. Urvashi Vaid, former director of the National Gay and Lesbian Task Force, conceded that "there are undeniably thousands of parents and siblings who have cared for their gay loved ones living with AIDS and HIV." She insisted, however, "that in the lives of most gay and bisexual men, this family never shows up." Amy Hoffman asserted, "With AIDS, nine times out of ten, it's the fake family who cleans up the shit." And Paul Monette castigated "the family sitting in green suburbia while the wasting son shuttles from friend to friend in a distant place, unembraced and disowned until the will is ready to be contested."[25]

Support for statements about the dereliction of family members comes from a 1995 study of both gay men and intravenous drug users diagnosed with AIDS in San Francisco. Members of both groups relied more on friends than on families for support. Other research, however, points to a more complicated reality. A study conducted between 1983 and 1986 in San Francisco reported that men who were both HIV-positive and symptomatic received more family support than did those who were HIV positive but asymptomatic. That finding suggested that "'when the chips are down,' barriers to social support from family of origin may be relaxed," or, in Robert Frost's more lyrical words, home is "the place where, when you have to go there, / They have to take you in.'"[26]

Like caregivers of people with dementia, family members caring for men with AIDS were overwhelmingly women. A few were wives and ex-wives. When Carol Lynn Pearson married Gerald in 1966, she knew he had had gay relationships in the past but believed faith and marriage could cure him. After eight years and the birth of four children, they divorced, and Gerald made a new life in the San Francisco gay community. When he phoned in the spring of 1984 to say he had AIDS, she became his primary caregiver, and he died in her home. Marion Winik met Tony Heubach at a New Orleans Mardi Gras weekend, when both were heavy drug users. Although he was gay and tested positive for HIV, they married and had two sons. Six years after the wedding, he was diagnosed with AIDS. The marriage gradually disintegrated, but Winik, too, provided care for several years. It was not an easy task. She worked at a job she hated because it provided health insurance. Heubach abused prescription medications and then began to take illicit drugs. When she threw him out of the house, his health rapidly declined, and she took him back and continued to nurse him, including administering the lethal injection he demanded.[27]

For many other women, an AIDS diagnosis represented a double shock. Elizabeth Cox and Keith Avedon had just celebrated their eleventh anniversary when Keith began to exhibit strange symptoms. Soon after he was diagnosed with AIDS, his sister told Cox that he previously had lived with a man. Later he divulged "the most devastating secret of his life": during their marriage he had had anonymous sex with men. "At that moment AIDS didn't matter to me," Cox wrote. "What he had done did. How did this fit into our life? Our life as I had seen it?" She quickly realized that AIDS was a far greater tragedy, however, and nursed him until his death.[28]

Like male partners, many wives were at high risk of contracting the disease. Marion Winik had shared hypodermic needles with her HIV-positive husband, and she continued to have sexual relations with him.

Contrary to her expectation, however, she tested negative. Elizabeth Cox at first refused to be tested, terrified that a positive result would mean her young son also had been infected. When she learned her test was negative, she "felt blessed and lucky—as if a hundred pounds had been lifted from my shoulders."[29]

Parents of people with AIDS represented another major source of care. Despite Paul Monette's caustic words about suburban families, he recalled that Roger Horwitz's parents "proved to be so heroic and so unflinching on the front lines that it's hard to recall when they were just the parents, benign in twilight." When the father praised the men's closeness, Monette commented, "It's a long way for a man to come who couldn't look me in the face for a year after Roger finally told him he was gay." Life-threatening disease similarly strengthened the bond between Fenton Johnson and the parents of his partner, Larry Rose. When Johnson arrived at their house the day after Rose told them he had tested positive for HIV, "the warmth and resonance of his parents' greeting made clear that my place in their eyes had been strengthened, both by what Larry had told them and by their understanding of the importance of a partner in facing such battles. . . . To his father I became, not just a friend of his son, but a genuine son-in-law. . . . Because of AIDS I became a member of the family." To be sure, an AIDS diagnosis could have the opposite effect. As a doctor in the AIDS clinic in a Northern California county hospital commented, "AIDS had the power to either break or mend a troubled relationship." When her friend Mike Riegle was close to death, Amy Hoffman informed his brother. He sent a scarf and pictures of his children but no note. Mike's parents had severed contact after he told them he was gay. In at least some cases, however, parents joined with partners and friends to extend the circle of care.[30]

Most parents who wrote reminiscences of the illness and death of their sons were mothers who had brought the men home to die. As in the case of Roger Horwitz's parents, AIDS often forced a reassessment of attitudes toward homosexuality. A clinical psychologist, Jean M. Baker, later berated herself for her reaction to her son's coming out. Gary had just completed his freshman year at Stanford when he told his parents he was gay. "In the immediate aftermath of Gary's devastating announcement," she wrote, "I cried every day. I was truly grieving." Recalling her feelings after his death, she wrote, "Now that my son had died, how strangely insignificant seemed the fact of his gayness. How difficult to believe I had ever thought his being gay was a tragedy. . . . The death of one's child is the ultimate tragedy." After her son's death, she became a gay rights advocate. But other equally devoted mothers inadvertently revealed lingering beliefs about their sons' personal responsibility for the disease. "Why is my son dying?" asked Beverly Barbo in the first page of her memoir, before answering, "Because he made some bad choices a few years ago, one of which resulted in the disease AIDS, and AIDS related cancer, Kaposi's Sarcoma is killing him." Ardath Rodale blamed the culture that urged her son to "enjoy sex to the fullest. . . . People were encouraged to experiment with the latest ideas. There were suggested positions for having sex that I never heard of before—never even imagined! People throughout the media winked an eye at, even openly approved of, multiple partners."[31]

Children figure prominently as caregivers to people with AIDS in Africa. In the United States, however, children were, in the words of two researchers, "an unlikely caregiving source for the AIDS population." In one well-documented case, the caregiver rather than the sufferer experienced a difficult homecoming. Alysia Abbott was one of the few women who described caring for a parent. She had lived with her father, Steve, in San Francisco since the age of two, when her mother was killed in a car accident. While she was spending her junior year in Paris, Steve told her that he had AIDS and that she needed to return. Back home, she felt out of step with her contemporaries and soon fell into despair. While her friends were in college or creating independent lives, she sat by her father's bed, accompanied him on depressing trips to the doctor, and prepared his food. A salesgirl job provided only a partial escape. When her father finally entered an inpatient hospice facility, she experienced a combination of sadness, guilt, and relief.[32]

Despite the sharp differences among the various groups of caregivers, they confronted many similar issues. One was the stigma surrounding AIDS. The cofounder and editor of *n+1*, a magazine of literature, culture, and politics, Marco Roth was in high school when he learned that his scientist father had AIDS and was expected to die within five years. "There was one more thing I knew, which had been impressed upon me," Marco later wrote. "I mustn't tell anyone about it." Paul Monette recalled that after Roger Horwitz's diagnosis, his brother demanded that their parents not be informed. "In fact, we couldn't tell anyone," Monette recalled. "A solo-practice lawyer, Horwitz feared his clients would flee as soon as word got out.[33]

Employment fears also kept Elizabeth Cox and her husband Keith Avedon from disclosing his condition to anyone but a few close friends and family. Their primary concern, however, was to protect their young son. "This catastrophic event in our lives goes unspoken so that our son won't lose a chance at getting into nursery school," Cox wrote, "so if Luke falls in the playground and is bleeding he won't be denied a hug." Secrecy exacerbated the loneliness of confronting a chronic, terminal disease. Cox and Avedon were "isolated and alone with our secret." As Avedon's illness entered its final stage, Cox's sense of isolation became almost unbearable. And concealment made her feel "confused," as if there was "something to be ashamed of."[34]

Caregivers also had to contend with the treatment loved ones received from the health care system. After rushing to New York's Lenox Hill Hospital to visit her desperately ill son, Jean M. Baker was shocked by a sign on the door instructing her to don a mask before entering his room. "The sign seemed to me to symbolize the stigma of AIDS," she wrote. In other cases, discrimination created access problems. Paul Monette had enormous difficulty in Los Angeles finding a nurse's aide willing to care for Roger Horwitz. Elizabeth Cox was startled to overhear a New York City doctor tell her husband just before an operation that he was lucky to have found a surgeon, because "most surgeons won't touch someone with AIDS."[35]

Some caregivers themselves worried about contamination. Years after her father died of AIDS in the early 1980s, Susan Bergman met the woman who had cared for him during his final months. Not knowing how the disease spread, the woman had kept his food on a separate shelf in her refrigerator and washed his clothes apart from her own. Bobbie Stasey's son Jim was diagnosed in 1988, after scientists understood the routes of transmission. Later she admitted that "there was a period of time when all the knowledge we had armed ourselves with could not dispel the fear that Jimmy would infect us." When he asked to taste her meal at a restaurant, she briefly panicked, terrified that the experts were wrong and that she, too, would become ill and die. Spouses and partners who continued to have sexual relations with HIV-positive people never could relinquish special precautions. "Sex used to imply abandon," Elizabeth Cox wrote. "Now it must involve restraint."[36]

Some aspects of the care relatives and friends delivered also aroused anxiety. Because the emergence of the AIDS epidemic coincided with the shift of the locus of care from hospitals to homes, the proportion of AIDS deaths occurring in hospitals steadily decreased. Enormous amounts of drugs and equipment accompanied people home. Elizabeth Cox complained after her husband's discharge: "Supplies were delivered over the weekend—carton after carton filled with bags and bottles and tubes and syringes. Bags of medicine have taken over the refrigerator. Cartons line the hall. Our home has been invaded by Keith's medicine." And Marco Roth remembered sitting next to his father on their white couch as he fed "AZT, DDI, and a dose of antibiotic, antifungal, and antiviral medicines in through the IV that ha[d] taken up permanent residence in our dining room."[37]

As the disease advanced, caregivers assumed increasing responsibility. Some tasks were relatively simple. Alysia Abbott helped her father count pills from the many vials adorning his bed stand. Bernard Cooper prepared herbs with Brian. Other caregivers performed complex medical and nursing tasks that were difficult to learn and that placed them at risk of infection. Bobbie Stasey took charge of cleaning and monitoring the catheter inserted into Jim's chest. She understood that if it became clotted, doctors would remove it, and Jim would have to undergo yet another procedure. She thus "watched it carefully" and "checked it many times a day."[38]

Because new crises could arise at any time, caregivers also made clinical assessments. During the many months her son lived at home, Barbara Peabody was constantly on the alert for new symptoms. "What does it all mean?" she asked, after noting that Peter had become "dull where he once was bright and observant" and that he rarely read serious books. Later she had other questions. Was his severe rectal pain from hemorrhoids or from another herpetic lesion? How could she tell whether neurological symptoms were seizures or the side effects of the medications that were supposed to prevent them? Could the small spot she found on his left shoulder be the first sign of Kaposi's sarcoma? When should she insist he see the doctor? She remained at home during the day and slept uneasily at night, "listening for every slight sound."[39]

Dignity

Researchers and policymakers commonly conceptualize caregiving in terms of specific tasks. That approach makes good sense. Gerontologists typically consider people to need care if they have functional limitations that prevent them from engaging in their daily activities. Almost by definition, then, caregivers are family members who enable patients to conduct those activities. Analyzing the specific chores that caregivers perform also has made it easier to recognize some of the ways caregiving has changed since the 1980s. And, as we have seen, some researchers have calculated the monetary value of particular tasks.

A few studies have found, however, that caregivers themselves are far less likely to concentrate on the chores they undertake than to emphasize the goals they wish to accomplish. Foremost among them is fostering their relatives' dignity. In the memoirs used in this study, that mission took various forms. Narratives of people with dementia typically included long sections describing the elders before disease struck, not only to emphasize what had been lost but also to assert that they were worthy of respect. When dementia still was mild, family members tried to respect their relatives' autonomy and encourage them to remain in control of their lives.[40]

As dementia progressed, caregivers found it more difficult to view their relatives as self-governing. Caregivers then increasingly tried to pretend that nothing had changed. Thus, they refused to enroll the elders in activities they previously would have considered demeaning, tried to keep their surroundings the same, and dressed them in the outfits they once might have chosen. Caregivers of people who had been professionals sought to create the illusion that they continued to command the respect they previously had enjoyed. Family members of women who had been housewives encouraged them to believe they still could make valuable contributions to the household.

Various scholars and researchers recently have asserted that people with dementia retain a sense of personal identity and that, rather than honoring the past, caregivers should emphasize and try to respond to the distinctive qualities they retain. Some caregivers in this study were able to appreciate the elders just as they were and enjoy their company. Novelist John Thorndike described the year he spent living with and caring for his father, Joseph J. Thorndike, who had been managing editor of *Life* and a founder of *American Heritage* and *Horizon* magazines. "I've grown closer to him," John wrote six months after arriving at his father's house. "It's brutal to watch your father slide into oblivion—and to imagine your own decline to come—but day after day I still want to be here in his house. I lay my hands on him, I listen to everything he says, and every morning I'm glad to see his face."[41]

Others learned to savor the present. Reeve Lindbergh's mother was Anne Morrow Lindbergh, the well-known author and the wife of the famous aviator. In 1989 she suffered a series of devastating strokes, and in 1999 Reeve brought her mother to live near her own house in Vermont. Fourteen months later, Reeve commented, "I am growing accustomed to having her alive, not the way she used to be, but exactly as she is. I am beginning to like our life together, right now. I don't understand this at all, but for the time being it makes me happy." Floyd Skloot, a poet, novelist, and nonfiction writer, was struggling to cope with serious brain damage when he realized his mother, who suffered from dementia, could teach him how to live within limitations. Watching the joy she found in her relationship with a man she met at her assisted living facility, Skloot wrote, "My mother . . . is still giving something vital back to me, reflecting the changes she endures with genuine grace, something of the changes I am trying to endure as well." Far more often, however, the writers focused on the past. Acting as custodians of the people they remembered, they mourned their losses and sought to repair them.[42]

Although family members of people with dementia had special concerns, they were not alone in emphasizing dignity and self-respect. Caregivers of people with various diagnoses focused on the need to promote patients' dignity when discussing intimate bodywork and the feelings of disgust it engendered. The topic of disgust recently has attracted large numbers of scholars and researchers from various fields. Many draw on the studies by psychologist Paul Rozin, who concluded that disgust arises from reminders of our animal nature, and especially of our mortality. Unlike the care literature, which emphasizes what individuals can gain from a confrontation with pain, vulnerability, and death, the disgust literature argues that humans cannot bear to contemplate their temporality for long. Disgust thus may weaken the desire to care. While care often reflects a sense of personal connection and can deepen and strengthen ties of interdependence, disgust propels aversion and avoidance.[43]

By its very nature, care for terminally ill people provides intimations of mortality. Closeness to death repelled Alan Shapiro when he visited his sister in the hospital shortly before the end: "The woman sitting on the edge of the bed, facing the door as I came in, was no one I'd ever seen before. . . . She seemed already dead in large part, her body taken from her replaced with this freakish stranger, her spirit reduced to creaturely distress so pure and unremitting that it made her cry out even as she slept." Shapiro knew he "ought to take her hand, massage her neck and forehead, touch her in some soothing way," but he "couldn't move." The two siblings had always been close, but their relationship had depended on intimate conversations, not physical contact. "To touch her now, I felt, would be to touch the brute, unvarnished fact of her dying; it would be to face her, as she was now, without a busy gloss of words between us. . . . Just to be with her now in silence, to take her hand, to touch her and not say anything, was to be intolerably present to her intolerable pain."[44]

Lauren Kessler's account highlights the magical thinking often considered a key ingredient of disgust. Although her mother suffered from dementia rather than a disease transmissible by germs, Kessler recoiled from contact with any object that had touched her. Kessler had not seen her mother during the nearly ten years her father had provided care in New York. When his health began to fail, Kessler offered to find a nursing home close to her home on the West Coast. She later wrote, "I cared for my mother on my own for exactly eighteen hours—I consulted my watch often—beginning when my husband and I picked her up at the airport . . . and ending when I signed her in at the care facility the next afternoon. I was terrified the entire time." After leaving her mother at the nursing home, Lauren "got out of there as fast as I could. When I got home I took the nightgown she had worn, the one I lent her, and put it in the trash. Just in case Alzheimer's was contagious."[45]

Caregivers also performed tasks that were fraught with disgust triggers. Personal care sometimes violated prohibitions against intimate physical contact between mothers and sons, fathers and daughters, sisters and brothers. "I never looked forward to helping my mother with her shower," wrote John Daniel. "She wasn't the least self-conscious about baring her body in my presence, but something in me shrank from it. To be with her in her nakedness seemed too intimate for a grown son."[46]

In addition, caregivers confronted bodily wastes. Now a novelist and short story writer, Laura Furman was a high school student when her mother battled ovarian cancer. "'Be careful where you step,'" an aunt instructed Laura, who was entering her mother's hospital room. The mother repeated the warning and then "turned her head so that I looked at the floor where there was a small puddle of vomit and blood." Laura left as soon as possible.[47]

Some caregivers had to handle body products. Like many people with advanced AIDS, poet Mark Doty's lover Wally Roberts suffered from diarrhea. "The first time I clean up a huge, particularly odorous mess," Doty wrote, "I feel an involuntary, physical sense of revulsion. I think I'm going to be sick." In *Patrimony*, Philip Roth wrote that when he brought his father home to recuperate from a serious operation, he complained about constipation for several days until the problem finally resolved with one large, explosive bowel movement. The smell reached Philip even before he entered the bathroom. In his typically exuberant style, he described what he saw:

> The shit was everywhere, smeared underfoot on the bathmat, running over the toilet bowl edge and, at the foot of the bowl, in a pile on the floor. It was splattered across the glass of the shower stall from which he'd just emerged, and the clothes discarded in the hallway were clotted with it. It was on the corner of the towel he had started to dry himself with. In this smallish bathroom, which was ordinarily mine, he had done his best to extricate himself from his mess alone, but as he was nearly blind and just up out of a hospital bed, in undressing himself and getting in the shower he had managed to spread the shit over everything. I saw that it was even on the tips of the bristles of my toothbrush hanging in the holder over the sink.[48]

William Ian Miller argued that disgust "does more than to register a simple aversion toward the objects of its focus. It degrades them in some way." The expression of disgust "always involves distance and superiority." But did the memoirists demean their relatives by describing the repulsion their bodies engendered? Some commentary suggests that they did. In his widely cited 2011 diatribe about the recent proliferation of confessional memoirs, Neil Genzlinger gave as an example one son's account of his mother's lingering death from cancer. The author "pummels us with the details," Genzlinger complained. He "strips her of any and all dignity by describing in voyeuristic detail her vomiting, diaper changes and such." Robert M. Adams singled out the passage by Philip Roth quoted above. Adams acknowledged that he "found it emotionally affecting to the point of pain." Nevertheless, "it was disturbing to have the old man's ultimate humiliation used as material for a mere book."[49]

The writers in this study, however, did not disclose unseemly details simply to expose their relatives to posthumous shame and humiliation. Some claimed to have gained something important from unavoidable contact with objects of disgust. "You clean up your father's shit because it has to be cleaned up," Philip Roth concluded, "but in the aftermath of cleaning it up, everything that's there to feel is felt as it never was before. It wasn't the first time that I'd understood this either: once you sidestep disgust and ignore nausea and plunge past those phobias that are fortified like taboos, there's an awful lot of life to cherish." Mark Doty assigned the title "Grace" to the chapter discussing Wally Roberts's incontinence. He wrote, "Shit is a new fact of life, and one I find myself thinking about; powerful, it interrupts every other interaction—no matter *what* else is going on, it stops while we clean up the shit. Like death, excrement is the body's undeniable assertion: *you will deal with me before all else, you will have no other priorities before me.*"[50]

Others presented intimate details to advance social action. The wife of a man with Alzheimer's disease and an advocate for other family members, Meryl Comer wanted policymakers and the general public to understand what daily, intimate care involved. Even a celebrated 2004 PBS documentary about the disease "never showed the real hands-on care." Thus, when the health correspondent for Jim Lehrer's PBS *NewsHour* asked Comer if she would be interviewed, she agreed to let a television crew into her house and even urged them to leave a camera so she could capture scenes when they were not around. "It was time to bring Alzheimer's disease out from behind the shadows of fear and stigma," she explained. "Living behind closed doors did not honor [her husband's] dignity." She not only described but also filmed an incident in which he had fallen after she had changed his diaper. "I let people see Harvey, totally helpless in his underwear and splayed on the floor, groaning unintelligibly."[51]

Moreover, memoirists emphasized their own extreme distress at the relatives' loss of dignity. "Poor Wally feels, I know, mortified at first," Doty commented. "He needs someone to wipe him, someone to clean him up; he has to let go of the privacy of the most personal of bodily functions, the most hidden." When Jean Baker learned that her son, who had AIDS, had been incontinent one night in the hospital, she felt his "humiliation with him, just one more indignity to suffer."[52]

If disgust pushed people away, it rarely extinguished all feelings of love. Adoring her mother, Laura Furman wrote that as soon as she fled the hospital room, she knew there was nowhere else she could be. And love sometimes helped to moderate feelings of disgust. "Because disgust critically involves things foreign to the self," wrote Paul Rozin and April E. Fallon, intimate relations, such as those between mother and child and lovers, "may weaken disgust by blurring the self-other distinction." Mark Doty's nausea "passes as quickly as it came. It's just Wally here in front of me, needing cleaning up, and he's easy to help." Although Fenton Johnson had not hesitated to become the lover of a man who was HIV-positive, he worried about his ability to provide care once Larry Rose was diagnosed with full-blown AIDS. When Rose suggested they live together, Johnson initially refused, fearful that Rose's needs would overwhelm his own life. But when Rose had an outbreak of boils during a trip to France, Johnson lovingly washed each with a warm cloth until it broke and then used a clean cloth to drain it. "In this gesture," he wrote, "I understood in some small way the love that motivates women and men who give their lives to the weak and ill. I understood the shallowness of my fears that I might abandon Larry once he grew sick. Now I wanted only to be with him and to care for him, for in caring for him I was caring for myself."[53]

In a few cases, feelings of revulsion reminded caregivers of family members' extreme vulnerability, heightening rather than blunting the desire to care. Duty alone could not explain the weekly visits novelist Mary Gordon paid to her mother and the assiduous way Gordon supervised her mother's care. Gordon "hated" her mother's body "except when I loved her for her helplessness. Then I loved her to the point of weeping unstoppable, wrenching tears."[54]

Many writers also had sought to minimize their relatives' feelings of shame. In some cases, that meant delegating the most intimate parts of personal care to outsiders, who had no emotional involvement. In other cases, memoirists performed the most unpleasant tasks themselves. Madeleine L'Engle cared for her mother, who had dementia, one summer with the help of neighborhood "girls." L'Engle explained why she had urged them to call her if her mother needed to be cleaned up at night. "Part of it was consideration for the girls. They are not being paid to take over the more unpleasant parts of nursing. Another reason is that I did not want anybody to witness the humiliation of my aristocratic mother."[55]

Finally, writers expressed respect for the ways relatives strove to defend their dignity in the face of physical deterioration. Richard Lischer explained that one reason his dying son tried to keep his most painful feelings to himself was that he could not bear his parents' grief. The other was that "with cancer some sort of physical overexposure—it doesn't deserve to be called 'intimacy'—becomes a daily occurrence, and it's disgusting. Wounds, night sweats, vomit, and horrible constipation—all of it must be cleansed, laundered, scrubbed, and suffered. If there's any dignity left, it won't occur in the body but in the patient's emotional life, where boundaries still count for something."[56]

Alan Shapiro had watched with awe as his sister Beth struggled after her bone marrow transplant, "not just to survive, but to preserve or discover within such terrible circumstances whatever dignity she could." At first he assumed she did so by thinking about her daughter or her work or her home when a nurse cleaned her after she had defecated in bed. Later he realized her physical pain was too overwhelming to allow her mind to wander. "Which is not say that she had lost her sense of dignity, for dignity, like pleasure, is relative to what the terms of life allow at any given moment. Her suffering had forced her temporarily to redraw the boundaries of her dignity, to shift it from its outward bodily manifestations onto something less dependent on what she couldn't now control." When she refused to use a bedpan or lowered the guardrail of her bed against a doctor's orders or spoke in the most matter-of-fact way about her soiled clothes, she "preserved what freedom, dignity, and personal autonomy she could find within such narrow straits." Her inability to hold on to the last shred of dignity shortly before she died cut him to the quick: "Struggling to pull herself up from the toilet seat, she finally had to call me in for help; there was no protection or defense against the disintegration of her dignity."[57]

Conclusion

Political scientist Nancy Fraser argues that decisions about whose needs should be deemed important are made "differently from culture to culture and from historical period to historical period." Although kin historically have been responsible for tending sick and dying people, the needs of family caregivers remained a private or domestic concern until the early 1980s. Three developments in those years enabled caregivers to begin to make political claims: the redefinition of senile dementia, rising anxiety about the diminishing supply of available family members, and the emergence of a terrifying epidemic creating new challenges for kin. The public policy response, however, has been minimal. The few supportive programs that exist provide little assistance and serve a tiny fragment of the population in need. The flourishing advice literature for caregivers may reduce stress but cannot alter the basic conditions of their lives.[58]

Although research on caregiving also has proliferated since the 1980s, most studies conceptualize caregiving as a series of tasks. The memoirs we have examined counter that instrumental approach by providing insight into how caregivers have understood and engaged in their work. Rather than focusing on the specific chores they undertook, family members emphasized the goals they wished to accomplish. Chief among them was sustaining relatives' dignity as their minds and bodies deteriorated. Family members of people with dementia viewed themselves as guardians of their relatives as they had been in the past. Those caring for people with AIDS portrayed them as uniquely precious human beings to nullify the stigma attached to the disease. And caregivers of people suffering from various illnesses sought to minimize the sense of shame they experienced when displaying symptoms commonly viewed as repulsive.

Many memoirs suggested, however, that the most serious threats to the dignity of patients came not from physical and mental decline but rather from the degrading treatment they received in health care institutions. The following chapter examines how the memoirists sought to protect relatives from those assaults in both hospitals and nursing homes.

5

The Shadow Workforce in Hospitals

and Nursing Homes

Although the vast caregiving literature focuses on patients at home, family care rarely ends when they enter medical institutions. Two researchers argue that kin deserve the title "shadow workforce," because they perform essential services in the fragmented and impersonal health care system. Above all, family members want to sustain relationships with their relatives in institutions, resist their objectification, and ameliorate their suffering. Those goals are not easy to achieve. In both hospitals and nursing homes, family members confront policies that seek to limit their presence and inhibit their involvement.[1]

"Five Minutes Are Up"

In 1980 the film critic Molly Haskell described seeing her gravely ill husband for the first time in an intensive care unit (ICU) as "an otherworldly experience." The unit "was like an airship, suspended in space, sterile because there was none of the ordinary signs or sounds of life, only whirring and clicking of machines surrounding mummy-like patients, each click signaling that death had been forestalled by another moment." She walked "along the small passageway, between two glass panes, where the patients four on the right, two on the left, were lined up side by side, with tubes of the most expensive machinery in the world reaching like tentacles into every orifice, and with their faces, peering out from oxygen masks, unrecognizable as to sex and age." Haskell concluded that "they weren't humans but cyborgs, half man-half machine, new arrivals on display from the planet of near death."[2]

Gerda Lerner, visiting her husband Carl in an ICU after his brain cancer surgery in 1972, learned that the other patient in the room recently had died. From waiting-room conversations, she heard about the deaths of other patients. And the atmosphere was redolent of mortality. "In the ICU death hovers on the ceiling," Lerner wrote, "a glittering, sterile, aluminum surface, forever reflecting light and light movements." To patients, those movements looked like "flickering candles, ghostly death signals." There was no night and no day. The following year another wife visited her husband in a unit that was so quiet it was like "a church or funeral home." His room "smelled like danger." The fluorescent light made "everything white, the dead waxen sheen of lilies."[3]

Six years after North Carolina Memorial Hospital in Chapel Hill established the first ICU in 1953, a survey found 238 units in short-term, private nonprofit hospitals. By 1965 the number of units had grown to 1,040. Although the first ICUs gathered critically ill patients together in one place and assigned special nurses to watch them full time, the units rarely contained more equipment than was available elsewhere in the hospital. In the 1960s, however, defibrillators, feeding tubes, and respirators began to fill ICUs. As the quoted comments suggest, the early ICUs were especially forbidding. Staff wore protective shoe covers and sometimes masks. Patients were heavily sedated. The massive equipment overwhelmed visitors.[4]

Strict visiting hours added to the sense of mystery and terror. Since the transformation of hospitals from welfare institutions to medical facilities at the turn of the twentieth century, middle- and upper-class families had enjoyed preferential access to hospitalized patients. In 1913, for example, New York's General Memorial Hospital for the Treatment of Cancer and Allied Diseases permitted visitors between 8:30 a.m. and 9:00 p.m. in private rooms but only between 1:30 and 3:00 p.m. in wards. Some hospitals allowed relatives and friends of private patients to rent adjacent rooms to sleep at night.

But no family members, regardless of background and hospital type, were permitted to remain long with patients in ICUs. A common assumption was that families were more likely to agitate than to comfort patients, and rest was considered especially important for those in ICUs. "The problem of visitors is a tedious and difficult one," noted a 1954 article in *Modern Hospital*. "Visitors must be the exception rather than the rule. Regulations must be passed and rigidly enforced." During the late 1960s and early 1970s, Elisabeth Kübler-Ross repeatedly criticized regulations that banished relatives who wished to hold deathbed vigils. Article after article contained a poignant description of a patient dying alone in an ICU while the family sat outside. Nevertheless, most hospitals continued to follow the 1962 recommendation of the Public Health Service that intensive care units limit visits to five minutes per hour.[5]

Tight security enforced strict regulations. Andrew H. Malcolm had just arrived from another state in 1991, when he tried to see his mother in an ICU at night. The unit's front door "was locked. No window. A 'No Unauthorized Entry' sign. Just a telephone that was silent when raised. . . . I could hear the faint rings behind the door. No answer. No Answer. No answer. No answer." A journalist who had written extensively about end-of-life care, Malcolm "knew ICUs; there was always someone there. Likely very busy. Probably checking me on a little TV camera, too. Yup, there it was up in the corner." Malcolm eventually gained entry that night, but many middle- and upper-class white family members experienced what less privileged relatives had long endured in hospitals. "Five minutes are up," a nurse informed Martha Weinman Lear in 1973. A prominent magazine writer, Lear had just flown from Europe and was seeing her husband, a well-known physician, for the first time after his massive heart attack.[6]

For many years, psychosocial theories about child development had encouraged both neonatal intensive care units (NICU) and pediatric intensive care units (PICU) to allow lengthy parental visits. Nevertheless, parents were not always satisfied. Gordon Livingston recalled that he and his wife were "horrified" by the limitations on visiting hours and the number of visitors in the Johns Hopkins Hospital PICU where their six-year-old son was dying in 1991.[7]

By that year nurses had begun to support family demands for more open visitation in ICUs for adults as well as children. As ICU gatekeepers, nurses had often confronted irate family members exiled to waiting rooms. Several had witnessed the desolation of the patients and families they forcibly separated. And several had personally experienced the pain inflicted by strict regulations. In addition, ICU nurses could now point to an important precedent. Husbands had campaigned for many years for the right to remain with their wives, first in labor rooms and then in delivery rooms. By the 1980s, men's presence was common in both units.[8]

One of the nurses' first tasks was to challenge the belief that families disturbed patients. A 1976 study had concluded that families had a negative physiological effect on patients. Nurses' studies reported that, on the contrary, family visits were more likely to lower rather than raise stress levels, whether measured by blood pressure, heart rate, or intracranial pressure. The benefits extended even to patients with neurologic injuries, who could not tolerate much stimulation. Nurses also focused on the needs of relatives, arguing that ICU staff had a responsibility to guard the well-being not just of patients but also of the people most intimately bound to them. In 2011 the American Association of Critical Care Nurses described family and friends as "partners in care" and called for unrestricted visitation policies in adult ICUs. The recent literature had shown that the unlimited "presence of a support person can improve communication, facilitate a better understanding of the patient, advance patient- and family-centered care, and enhance staff satisfaction."[9]

Another champion of open visitation was Dr. Donald Berwick, a Harvard pediatrician and professor as well as president and CEO of the Institute for Healthcare Improvement (he later was administrator of the Center for Medicare and Medicaid Services). In 2003 Berwick challenged hospitals to institute totally unrestricted visiting hours in the ICU for a period of two months and then evaluate the results. The following year he published an article in the *Journal of the American Medical Association* entitled "Restricted Visiting Hours in ICUs: Time to Change?" He, too, cited the accumulating research, arguing that restricted ICU visiting was "neither caring, compassionate, nor necessary." In 2010 Berwick again addressed the topic in a Yale School of Medicine graduation speech. Shortly before coming to Yale, he had received a letter from a woman whose physician husband had been a patient in a Pennsylvania hospital following a cerebral bleed. "My issue," she wrote, "is that I was denied access to my husband except for very strict visiting, four times a day for 30 minutes, and that my husband was hospitalized behind a locked door. My husband and I were rarely separated except for work. He wanted me present in the ICU, and he challenged the ICU nurse and MD saying, 'She is not a visitor, she is my wife.' But it made no difference. My husband was in the ICU for eight days out of his last 16 days alive, and there were a lot of missed opportunities for us." She concluded, "I feel that it was a very cruel thing that was done to us."[10]

Efforts to open ICU doors have enjoyed considerable success. The various surveys of visitation policies since the 1980s focus on different groups of hospitals and ask different questions. Nevertheless, it is clear that although change has been slow, the trend has been toward more flexible visitation. That has not pleased everyone. Although many nurses spearheaded efforts to reform rigid visitation regimes, others expressed dismay at the disappearance of familiar restrictions. Between 1998 and 2012, ten nursing blogs debated the issue of open visitation. Nurses opposed to that reform were greatly overrepresented among the contributors. More than half of nurses support open visitation. Twenty-seven (16%) of the 168 nurses who posted comments either were ambivalent or simply offered advice. Of the other 141 contributors, 109 (77%) opposed change. Those nurses also tended to express their views with special vehemence. While proponents of open admission typically presented their arguments in a straightforward, unemotional manner, many opponents used strong, occasionally vitriolic, language. Open visitation, they contended, was "ludicrous," "horrendous," a "fad," "nuts," and a "truly bad idea." The consequences had been "disastrous." Several contributors either had left ICU nursing or vowed to do so as soon as possible.[11]

Witnessing Resuscitation Efforts

Sandra M. Gilbert, a distinguished poet and professor of English at the University of California–Davis, filed a wrongful death suit after her sixty-year-old husband Elliott Gilbert, the chair of the same department, died in 1991 following routine surgery for prostate cancer. When his heart stopped, the doctors tried to resuscitate him. Sandra was neither informed of his condition nor invited to be with him. In a letter she later imagined sending his surgeon, she charged that he may have eliminated Elliott's last chance of life. She noted that "survivors of 'near-death experiences' are often in some sense 'called back' by loved ones." But above all, she wished she and her daughters had "been there with him, there when he was forced through the enormous wall between what we know and what we don't know, there to try to comfort him as he was dragged away from us." "Who," she asked, "administered 'Last Rites' to my husband? What were his final words? . . . Did you hear them, or did some nurse listen to them? Did she turn away, ignoring what he said? Or did she take his hand and console him?" Other questions continued to haunt her: "Was there a moment when he realized what was happening, a moment of transition and recognition? Was he frightened? Was he resigned? Did he ask for me? Did he remember me? Did he remember *himself*?" As she had learned from nineteenth-century literature, the final moment is "a majestic one in every life" and family members needed to be there.[12]

Although some resuscitation efforts occur in ICUs, the great majority take place in emergency rooms. Pressure for family presence at resuscitative attempts arose at the same time as the drive for more lenient ICU visitation and reflected similar concerns, but the campaigns differed in two significant ways. Doctors rather than nurses controlled entry to resuscitation rooms and thus played major roles in determining hospital policy. In addition, open ICU policies often specified that families could be removed during procedures. By definition, resuscitation efforts are procedures with extremely high stakes. Although television shows suggest that the success rate is high, very few people who undergo CPR survive. Most of those who do either die before they can leave the hospital or experience very serious functional limitations after discharge.[13]

Attempts to revive dying patients began as early as the 1800s but increased dramatically after 1962, when doctors agreed that the best technique was cardiopulmonary resuscitation (CPR), which involves opening the airways, mouth-to-mouth ventilation, and chest compression. Although most efforts failed, advocates argued that lay people could learn to perform the procedure and that it could benefit everyone who suffered a cardiac arrest. In the mid-1970s, many communities integrated CPR with their emergency care systems. New guidelines continued to emphasize the immediate steps bystanders could take but also urged them to summon medical assistance. Ambulances outfitted with drug therapies, defibrillators, and intravenous pumps rushed patients to hospital emergency rooms, where doctors continued the efforts while families waited outside. "A resuscitative effort following a sudden collapse," writes sociologist Stefan Timmermans, has had "all the properties of a feared technological death with abandonment in the hospital."[14]

The opening salvo in the campaign to allow family presence during CPR efforts occurred in 1982, when Hank Post, the chaplain of W. E. Foote Memorial Hospital in Jackson, Michigan, attempted to honor the wishes of two women whose husbands were about to undergo CPR. The first was the wife of Craig Scott, a state trooper who had been shot in the back by the driver of a stolen car. After repeated requests from Post, the doctors finally allowed her to watch. The second case also involved the wife of a state trooper. Bill Sherman had suffered a cardiac arrest shortly after arriving at the hospital complaining of chest pains. When his wife Alice learned he had been rushed to a trauma room, she insisted on following him. Again Post conveyed the request to the doctors, who finally consented to Alice's presence, though just for a few minutes. Post later recalled her saying, "I know he's dying. I'm just glad I could tell him I love him before he dies. And I wanted to make sure that everything possible was being done for him." Soon after that incident, the hospital instituted a program allowing selected family members to watch resuscitation efforts. Most staff members who were interviewed supported family presence, but a few indicated that it increased stress by making the patient appear "more human."[15]

Although families continued to demand entry to resuscitation rooms throughout the country, the issue did not again capture national attention until 1993, when the Emergency Nurses Association (ENA) passed a resolution declaring that family members had a right to attend resuscitation efforts and urging hospitals to give them the option of doing so. The following year an emergency room nurse challenged the policy of the major public facility in Dallas, Texas. Theresa A. Meyers was on duty at Parkland Hospital and Health System, when Donnie Hoyt, a fourteen-year-old boy, arrived after falling from a tree and lacerating his liver. He soon was rushed to the ICU. When the parents showed up, Meyers took them to the unit, only to be told they could not enter because Donnie was receiving CPR. She then asked the surgeon for permission to allow them to watch. After receiving reluctant approval, Meyers led the parents into the room. "We stood at the bedside," Meyers later wrote, "and the mother and father talked to their son. The father apologized for an argument they'd had the day before, and both parents told their son how much they loved him and how good he was." After his death, the parents thanked the doctor for his efforts on the boy's behalf. "The next few weeks were uncomfortable for me," Meyers continued. "Some powerful people in the institution felt I had crossed the professional line and should be fired."[16]

Nevertheless, the hospital agreed to institute a pilot program to allow family presence at resuscitation efforts and asked Meyers and a few colleagues to evaluate it. Even before the results were published, stories about the study began to appear in the national media. A 1998 *Redbook* article advised parents how to obtain permission to watch children's CPR. Extensive media coverage also followed the report of the study in the February 2000 issue of the *American Journal of Nursing*, encouraging more relatives to demand entry to resuscitation areas. According to Meyers and her coauthors, most family members who had observed resuscitative attempts were pleased they had done so and would do so again. Guidelines published by the American Heart Association a few months later advocated family-witnessed resuscitation.[17]

But acceptance of family attendance at CPR was far from universal. Another 2000 article noted that trauma surgeons had responded to the concept of family presence at resuscitation with "considerable skepticism and incredulity." A research team led by R. Stephen Smith, a trauma surgeon and professor at the University of Kansas School of Medicine in Wichita, had surveyed the opinions of members of both the ENA and the American Association for the Surgery of Trauma (AAST). Although the overwhelming majority of respondents from the two groups believed that family presence during resuscitation was inappropriate, AAST members were far more likely than ENA members to believe that family presence interfered with patient care and increased physician stress. ENA members were more likely to believe that family members had a right to observe resuscitation. The article also listed the respondents' major concerns. Because guns were widely available in the United States and few emergency rooms had metal detectors, irate relatives permitted to enter resuscitation areas easily could harm both patients and team members. Like some nurses opposed to open ICU visitation, many doctors also stressed the need to protect families. Resuscitation was such a gruesome procedure that it easily could inflict permanent psychological harm on relatives who observed it.[18]

Finally, doctors argued that family members could distract the medical team. The authors noted with approval the Federal Aviation Administration's "sterile cockpit rules," which prohibited crew members from engaging in nonessential activities during crucial stages of a flight. "The resuscitation of a critically injured trauma patients and the operation of a complex aircraft have many similarities," the article stated. "Both tasks require the assimilation of a large quantity of data in a short period of time and quick decision-making based on the information at hand." In comparing themselves to airline pilots, those doctors made it clear that they viewed their work solely as a set of technical tasks, unrelated to the singular aspects of patients' lives.[19]

Although subsequent research has allayed those concerns, most studies have been small and observational. Considerable attention thus has focused on a large French study reported in the *New England Journal of Medicine* in 2013. Relatives who witnessed CPR had fewer symptoms of anxiety and depression than others, and family presence had no effect on patient survival. But controversy continues to surround the issue. Although many professional organizations now support family presence at resuscitative efforts, only 10 percent of hospitals have written policies to allow relatives to observe the procedures.[20]

Social Status

In February 2014, Dr. Arnold Relman, a distinguished physician and former medical editor, wrote in the *New York Review of Books* about the excellent medical care he received at Massachusetts General Hospital after falling down a flight of stairs and suffering many life-threatening injuries. A few months later, the journal published a letter from a physician in Puerto Rico, expressing gratitude for Relman's recovery but also pointing out that he had failed to mention the special privileges he undoubtedly had enjoyed: "In the Massachusetts General Hospital emergency room someone is bound to have said that Dr. Relman had arrived." In reply, Relman wrote that his treatment "would have been pretty much the same in the emergency room, but probably not thereafter, in the intensive care unit." The staff "allowed members of my family (particularly the physicians in the family) to stay at my bedside after visiting hours." Here he emphasized the medical help they provided; his previous letter had highlighted the comfort they bestowed in alien surroundings.[21]

Even without Dr. Relman's eminence, well-educated and affluent patients may often receive special consideration. Various researchers conclude that hospital staff have enormous discretion in enforcing regulations in both ICUs and emergency rooms and that practice thus often diverges sharply from policy. One study found that ICU nurses often made the decisions about granting exceptions "on the basis of individual intuition and experience, rather than any consistent plan or guidelines." An account of an emergency room noted that nurses routinely specify that only "selected" families should be allowed to observe CPR efforts. One nurse observed that she had been able to invite next of kin to witness resuscitation attempts because she practiced in a Canadian town with a population of ten thousand. "I can be 'selective,'" she wrote, "because someone almost always knows the patient or family." A physician at W. E. Foote Hospital in Michigan reported that staff members do a "quick read" to determine which family members should be permitted to enter resuscitation sites.

And a nurse in Greenville, Kentucky, stressed the need for staff to rely on their "gut" feelings. Nurses who depend on "gut" feelings and "intuition and experience" may be especially lenient toward families with high social status.[22]

Nevertheless, some have continued to tell stories of painful separation. One might have expected Kay Redfield Jamison and Richard Wyatt to have been able to dictate their own terms in 2002 when Wyatt was dying at George Washington University Hospital. He was chief of the neuropsychiatry branch of the National Institute of Mental Health; Jamison was a professor of psychiatry at the Johns Hopkins School of Medicine. Nevertheless, a nurse demanded that Jamison leave. Later she realized she had experienced "the primitive distress of an animal being taken from its dying mate."[23]

Even units with flexible visitation policies typically excluded families during shift changes, when nurses and doctors exchanged confidential patient information. Vicki Forman was very familiar with the health care system by the time she sat by her tiny son in an NICU on an evening in 2000. When she was twenty-three weeks pregnant, she had gone into labor and given birth to twins, each weighing less than a pound. Although she had begged the doctors not to try to keep them alive, they had insisted on resuscitation. Forman's daughter Ellie died after a few days, but her son Ethan survived with an array of life-threatening disabilities. Recently he had been transferred to a large urban hospital for an operation to try to save his eyesight. Forman wrote, "I sat and rocked him, tried to feed him, then held a syringe of formula and watched the milky liquid sling through the tube into his nose, all this through a veil of tears. . . . I watched the clock and waited for the retinologist. At ten to seven, a nurse approached me. 'Mrs. Forman? I'm sorry . . .' I looked at the clock and realized I had committed a cardinal sin: I was bedside during shift change." The nurse demanded that Forman leave "even though I had hardly arrived, even though I was clutching my son and in tears about his fate."[24]

"Put the Parent in a Nursing Home?"

Although nursing homes evoke widespread anxiety, they are central to the long-term care system, and many family members consider resorting to them at some point. The facilities arose in the wake of the 1935 Social Security Act. Seeking to curtail the use of almshouses, that law stipulated that blind and needy people could receive aid only if they lived at home or in private institutions. By the early 1950s, fourteen thousand nursing homes were scattered throughout the country; most were small, private facilities. The almshouse population had plunged by nearly half, from 135,000 to 72,000 since the early 1930s. Observers soon reported, however, that many problems of the almshouse had been transferred to nursing homes. Although most residents suffered from serious chronic conditions, medical attention was sparse and inadequate. Buildings were dilapidated and often unsanitary.[25]

The 1965 establishment of Medicare and Medicaid dramatically increased public funding for nursing homes and thus their numbers. Because those programs also imposed regulations that small, "mom and pop" homes had difficulty meeting, larger, more medically oriented institutions began to emerge. Following repeated exposés of abusive conditions, the US Senate Special Committee on Aging held a series of hearings between 1963 and 1974, leading to the reform of both federal and state regulations. Nevertheless, a 1986 report by the Institute of Medicine concluded that a high proportion of nursing home residents received "shockingly deficient care." The 1987 Nursing Home Reform Act addressed some, but by no means all, of the problems.[26]

Today, six thousand US nursing homes serve a total of 1.4 million residents. Although the majority are for-profit, the government pays the bill. Medicaid is the primary funding source, covering 63 percent of residents. Some enter facilities as Medicaid beneficiaries; others qualify for Medicaid after exhausting their resources. Although many older Americans assume that Medicare covers nursing home stays, that program is tilted toward acute care and pays for less than 15 percent of the residents. Grave concerns about quality of care persist. In 2008 state surveyors found that 25.6 percent of nursing homes had deficiencies that harmed residents or placed them in immediate jeopardy. Homes with the highest proportion of residents financed by Medicaid tend to give the worst care.[27]

A combination of economics and humanitarianism has spurred attempts to reduce the size of the nursing home population. Although Medicaid remains oriented toward institutions, the proportion of the program's spending on home- and community-based care more than doubled between 1995 and 2007. Another alternative to nursing homes is assisted living facilities, which private groups and individuals began to establish in the mid-1980s.

The goal was to grant residents more autonomy than they could have in nursing homes and provide less institutional surroundings. By 2007 more than one thousand assisted living facilities were in operation.[28]

Nevertheless, nursing home care often remains the only option. Despite recent funding increases, public home- and community-based services are not uniformly available. Those that exist have long waiting lists. And many families have too much money to qualify for public services but too little to pay privately. The average hourly rate of a private home health aide is $21. For adult day care, the average daily rate is $70. Assisted living costs on average $3,550 a month, and most facilities discharge residents who are considered too disabled.[29]

If some public policies and private initiatives seek to keep people out of nursing homes, the caregiving discourse may have the opposite effect, especially for those suffering from dementia. Approximately half of nursing home residents have some form of cognitive impairment; 14 percent have a diagnosis of Alzheimer's disease. Over and over, health professionals, books, websites, and support groups remind family members of the following points: Caregivers' physical and mental health is as important as that of their relatives. Too much stress can lead to "burnout," making further home care impossible. Family members who place relatives with dementia in nursing homes are not "failures" and should not feel guilty. Because nursing homes employ trained and skilled staff, they can offer the most appropriate care and keep people with advanced disease safer than they could be at home. Rather than "dumping" relatives into nursing homes, most Americans consider institutionalization only as a last resort. But virtually all people with dementia will need to enter nursing homes at some point. Because beds are scarce and people with dementia can adjust to nursing home care better before they reach the most advanced stages of their disease, family members should begin to investigate possible facilities early in the disease course.[30]

Of the twenty-three memoirists used in this study who wrote about people with dementia, nineteen noted that they had considered nursing home placement. Like other relatives of people with dementia, most initially had refused to do so. (Although a growing number of people now enter nursing homes for short-term rehabilitation, the writers examined here contemplated placement for stays that would end only with the patient's death.) "Put the parent in a nursing home? It never occurred to me," wrote Elinor Fuchs, a professor at the Yale Drama School, describing the early years of caring for her mother, Lil. Elinor never could have anticipated that she would spend a decade as a dutiful daughter. After the end of her marriage, Lil had left Elinor with her grandparents to launch a career as a businesswoman. Although she eventually reunited with her daughter, Lil continued traveling throughout the Middle East and Asia, selling motor tools and automotive parts to foreign governments. She assumed Elinor could raise herself. But during the ten years following her mother's diagnosis of Alzheimer's disease, Elinor discovered that "taking care of" might be "as good as being taken care of." She traveled regularly from New York to Washington and carefully supervised her mother's care by phone at other times. She eventually placed Lil in a nursing home, but only near the end of her life, after all other options had been exhausted.[31]

In most cases, recommendations for nursing home placement first came from professionals. John Thorndike recalled that after his father's dementia diagnosis, the doctor "assumed that sooner or later I'd find it too difficult to look after my father at home, and we'd have to move him." Other writers had received encouragement from social workers, home health aides, friends, and other family members to place a relative in a nursing home.[32]

But, like Elinor Fuchs, most writers were not easily convinced that institutionalization was a good idea. Some stressed their responsibility to care for their own. Although Linda McK. Stewart's husband Jack had retired from his editorial position at the *New York Times*, he was enjoying freelance work when he suddenly showed signs of advanced Alzheimer's disease. Linda later wrote that, despite the burdens of tending him, handing over his care to an institution "was a concept I was incapable of accepting." John Daniel declared, "I hate that America is a society of foster homes and nursing homes and retirement towers. I hate that we farm out our elders when they aren't useful anymore and can no longer do for themselves and begin to intrude on our precious convenience." He had hoped to be different.[33]

Because the narrative writers were overwhelmingly middle-class, they typically were able to pay privately for nursing home care for at least some period from the relatives' long-term care insurance or personal funds. None was restricted to a Medicaid facility at the outset. In addition, all were well aware of the poor quality of the average nursing home when they embarked on the search for a place for their relative. Nevertheless, what they discovered appalled them. Whether because they believed that good care could protect their relatives from the worst ravages of the disease, or because they did not want to face what advanced dementia often looked like, the sight of the residents was especially disturbing. Judith Levine visited two well-regarded nursing homes in Manhattan. "They win awards," she wrote. "They devise their policies from up-to-date research on dementia, train their staffs and evaluate the 'outcomes' of their programs conscientiously." But in both facilities she found many residents who "loll in wheelchairs, uncommunicative and, at least when we were there, uncommunicated with." Elinor Fuchs toured the two most highly recommended nursing homes in Washington, D.C. "I scratched the first one off the list as soon as I got there. I couldn't bear the sight of old folks in wheelchairs watching TV at noon, eyes glazed, chins hanging slack. From the stench I guessed that most of them were drenched in urine. No one seemed to regard this as a problem." She "reeled back, choking, and fled." The second, reputed to have the best program for people with dementia "was a kindergarten wrapped in a prison."[34]

Family members also recoiled from the idea of informing their relatives that they would have to leave home. John Daniel, for example, "couldn't begin to imagine telling [his mother] that she had to go." Elizabeth Cohen, a single mother and reporter, had been caring for both an infant and her father for several months when she tried to convince her father that entering a nursing home might be better than remaining alone in her house all day. In response, he pointed to his temple, cocked his finger like a pistol, and said, "This is where I want to stick a bullet if it comes to that." (Such a response probably was not unusual. A 1997 study found that 30 percent of elderly people would rather die than move permanently into a nursing home.)[35]

But many family members also had compelling reasons to consider nursing homes. Linda McK. Stewart phoned her son Mark whenever crises arose with her husband. Mark came right away, but "after half a dozen such SOS calls, it was evident that something profound had to change. There were days when Mark had to be away on business. What then?" She decided to explore the nursing homes in her area.[36]

Other family members were forced to withdraw relatives from assisted living facilities. Floyd Skloot's mother needed more care and supervision than the staff could provide. Elinor Fuchs realized that her mother no longer could participate in the activities that previously had made the facility attractive. And Eleanor Cooney learned that the staff could not deal with her mother's agitation and combativeness and that she scared the other residents.[37]

Other arrangements also unraveled. A majority of family members had hired aides to provide care at home, but the relatives hated being treated like children with babysitters, the family members disapproved of the care aides provided, and most aides did not remain long on the job. Adult day care programs had still other problems. Some of those enrolled in the programs regarded the activities as too demeaning and refused to return. Aaron Alterra had been delighted to find a program for his wife that gave him a few hours of relief each week. After a year, however, the director told him that his wife required too much assistance and no longer could attend.[38]

Nursing home admission also made financial sense. Most memoirists who had relied on aides and attendants had paid for them out of pocket. As the assets of the ill person gradually dwindled, nursing home admission began to look more attractive. (Although the annual cost was prohibitive for most families, residents could apply for Medicaid after exhausting their resources.) When Marion Roach and her sister realized that their mother no longer could live alone in her house, they moved her to a nearby apartment. By borrowing against the house, they were able to pay the rent and also afford around-the-clock care from various aides. Many people told them that a nursing home would be cheaper, but Marion and her sister "couldn't stand" that idea. "We decided to do everything else before even considering such a placement," Marion recalled. After a year, however, the money was nearly gone. When the director of a nursing home phoned to say he had an opening, the sisters reluctantly enrolled their mother.[39]

Finally, family members pointed to evidence that the ailing relative had reached an advanced stage of dementia. That argument received the approval of advice givers, but it often ignited family conflict. We saw in chapter 4 that Barry Petersen adhered closely to the biomedical model of Alzheimer's disease, presenting his wife Jan as a case study. By the time he decided to place her in an institution, he was convinced she had reached the sixth of the seven stages. So when he wrote to inform family and friends of his plan and that she had become too disabled to live at home, he assumed they would agree. Instead, they accused him of betrayal. His response was to continue to invoke expert advice, organizing a meeting and inviting a social worker to speak. The social worker arrived "with charts and pictures and explained in graphic and uncompromising detail how Alzheimer's attacks, physically alters, and destroys the brain. . . . She was teaching her version of Alzheimer's 101, because if you do not know The Disease and have not lived with it for years or decades, it can fool with ease." Her lecture persuaded some, though not all, of Jan's friends and family that Petersen had made the right decision.[40]

Judith Levine, by contrast, had read the emerging literature on the persistent "personhood" of people with dementia and drew on that theory to understand the progression of her father's Alzheimer's. She ridiculed the mental tests her mother trusted. "Mom organizes and substantiates her own observations of Dad's slide with expert assessments," she wrote. Determined to resist "the medical standardization of dementia," Judith tossed "away the chart of stages" and took note of what was "stable in Dad, even flourishing." When her mother announced that she had been dating another man, Judith feared that new relationship with a "fully function-ing peer" made her husband's deficits appear larger than they actually were. The conflict escalated when the mother said she wanted to place her husband in a nursing home. Judith accompanied her mother on tours of possible facilities but insisted that her father still loved his home and could receive good care there. She thus protested when her mother began the process of institutionalization by applying for Medicaid and arranging the assessments the facilities demanded. At the end of the memoir, the mother went to live with her boyfriend, leaving her husband in the apart-ment with full-time aides. The issue of nursing home placement remained unresolved.[41]

In several instances, family members still were debating nursing home placement when a specific event suddenly precipitated action. An aide quit or went on vacation; the relative's health sharply deteriorated; or, as in the case of Marion Roach, a nursing home director phoned to say a room was available. But sometimes it was difficult to determine just what had forced the decision. Rachel Hadas, the author of numerous works of poetry and a professor at Rutgers University, Newark, described her years caring for her husband George, who had been a composer, writer, and professor of music at Columbia University. As dementia descended, he gradually ceased virtu-ally all activity and became increasingly quiet. Hadas realized, "If there was one reason I decided that I could no longer live with George, that coor-

dinating his care had gone from arduous and unrewarding routing to unbearable pain, that reason was the grinding loneliness imposed by his silence, the almost unbroken silence." But long after she began to investigate
available places and make the necessary financial arrangements, she wondered when she should force him to leave. "When our interests and needs
no longer coincided, what was the best thing for both of us? For him?
For me? For our son? When George no longer taught, composed, played the
piano, read, wrote? When he had almost completely ceased smiling,
speaking? When he was sleeping fourteen hours a day?" In retrospect, she
realized that both the death of a woman she had known and a dinner conversation with another caregiver after the memorial service had affected
her. "I lay awake that night, and for reasons I do not know, but which felt
then and still feel now connected with that memorial service and that dinner," she recalled, "I crossed a line in my mind. This life I was living was too
hard, and it could easily go on, getting gradually harder for decades. I was
exhausted and lonely. George was less and less present." Soon afterward,
she moved him to a nursing home.[42]

Of course, individual preferences alone could not determine the course
of action. Elizabeth Cooney began to search for a suitable nursing home
immediately after her mother's discharge from an assisted living facility.
Because Cooney lived in a small northern California town, she assumed
she would not find the same poor quality of care she knew existed in major
metropolitan areas. She quickly realized, however, that wherever she put
her mother, "she'll be in hell. And so will I." Cooney eliminated the first
two possibilities as unbearably grim. Her third visit was to "Dunwood Oaks,"
an unglamorous small-town nursing home that she never had considered
even the remotest option. Nevertheless, she decided it would be her mother's
next home. But Dunwood Oaks administrators learned about the mother's
behavior in assisted living and rejected her application. Cooney next explored a place four hours away in Davis, again, by no means a "snake-pit," but
"the fluorescently lit institutional atmosphere" and the "drooling" residents
dismayed her. Because Dunwood Oaks phoned to say they would take the
mother on a two-week trial basis, she told the Davis facility to offer the bed
to someone else. Then Dunwood Oaks rescinded the offer.[43]

Although Cooney previously had dismissed a Santa Rosa facility as too
far away, she now reconsidered. In comparison with the dismal places
she had seen, this one seemed somewhat attractive. The waiting list was

formidable, however, and Cooney feared that if a bed opened, the facility would reject her mother after an evaluation. A friend mentioned "a small, very exclusive residence for old ladies" that clearly would be unable to handle her mother. Desperate, Cooney consulted the Yellow Pages and found a nursing home that advertised a specialized Alzheimer's unit. "I call," she wrote. "Instant brick wall: sorry, no room at the inn. But if you'd care to leave your name and number . . ." With the help of an advocacy group for caregivers, Cooney finally learned of a vacancy at Sheffield House in Vacaville and decided to take her mother there, sight unseen.[44]

Most family members experienced leaving a relative at a nursing home as a brutal act, especially when the relative could comprehend what was happening. Elinor Fuchs brought her mother, Lil, to a facility in the morning and then left for a few hours to take care of other affairs. Returning in the afternoon, she found her mother in her room, surrounded by nurses doing an intake examination "She is stripped naked and slowly being rotated. They note every discoloration or crack in the skin, the way my car dealer inspects my car before a tune-up: both want to protect themselves from lawsuits. The nurses ask Lil to lift her arms, spread her legs, bend over. Mother tries to smile and laugh, but tears run down her face. She understands, I think, that she has become a 'case.'" Eleanor Cooney believed her mother gradually adjusted to life at Sheffield House but never forgave her daughter for sending her there. "The bitterest, bitterest sadness for me," Cooney wrote, "is knowing that she believed I betrayed and abandoned her." A few months after her mother's admission, Cooney found a photograph of herself, ripped in half.[45]

Marion Roach was one of the few caregivers who discovered that institutionalization could benefit residents. Within three months of admission to a nursing home, her mother had regained 20 percent of her speech. Because she engaged in various activities, she no longer was lonely. And, for the first time in months, she recognized her daughter: "She knew I was someone who loved her and someone whom she loved," Roach wrote. "She'd ask me how I was. Not much more, but that was a lot." Sue Miller had the opposite, and far more common, experience. In an assisted living facility, her father's decline had been "slow, but steady." After his transfer to a nursing home, the pace accelerated. "Within days, almost literally before my eyes," she recalled, "he became radically more demented." Similarly, Lucette Lagnado, an Egyptian-born reporter for the *Wall Street*

Journal, believed that because her mother "couldn't cope with the harshness of her new surroundings," she "rapidly deteriorated." Whenever Lucette visited the nursing home, she found her mother "slumped in her wheelchair, fast asleep. She spoke to no one and barely ate or drank." Lucette concluded, "My mother had lost any semblance of an identity; she was simply a woman against a wall."[46]

Popular advice books encourage caregivers to remain closely connected to relatives in nursing homes, visiting and telephoning frequently, filling the rooms with personal items, showing interest in the facilities, and celebrating birthdays and holidays together. Like most other family members, the narrative writers in this study tried to heed that advice. Because Sue Miller found her father's room stripped of all the personal items he had kept in the assisted living facility, she tried to have his favorite chair quickly recovered with a fire-retardant fabric to conform to the nursing home's regulations.[47]

Although studies indicate that efforts such as those may persuade staff members to bestow more attentive care, there clearly are limits to what family members can accomplish. *The 36-Hour Day* informs families that when abuse occurs, they can contact an Alzheimer's Association chapter or the local nursing home ombudsman; in extreme cases, families can send reports to the state nursing home inspector's office. Otherwise, the guide urges, relatives should proceed cautiously: "The director of an excellent home suggests that you avoid complaints and do all that you can to establish a friendly relationship with the staff. This may mean a compromise on your part, but it may well encourage their cooperation."[48]

The narrative writers in this study quickly discovered the truth of that advice. When Sue Miller protested her father's care, "everyone agreed with me, about everything. The social worker even ran a special program for the staff as a result of my speaking up. . . . But after this the head nurse was chillier to him than ever. . . . I wondered then what my stepping forward on his behalf had cost him." Lucette Lagnado felt "powerless to make any changes" in the miserable treatment her mother received. "The nursing home tended to dismiss whatever complaints I made because I was 'the daughter' and they expected daughters to be difficult and had learned to tune them out and to keep doing exactly what they were doing." And Virginia Stem Owens, a novelist who moved from Kansas to Texas to be close to her mother, "tried to make as few complaints as possible" after placing her in a facility. As in any institution, she concluded, "you learn to spend your credit carefully."[49]

Conclusion

"Hospital spaces and schedules are designed to treat diseases," writes sociologist Arthur W. Frank. "They do not accommodate people trying to sustain relationships while illness is tearing apart their lives. When medical staff need assistance, they expect the caregiver to be on call; otherwise he or she is a visitor." Much has changed since Elisabeth Kübler-Ross castigated hospitals for banishing kin when death was imminent. A growing number of institutions have removed the most restrictive visitation regulations in intensive care units, and some allow family presence at resuscitation attempts. Nevertheless, many doctors and nurses continue to view families as impediments to good care. Although nurses and doctors may be more likely to make exceptions for affluent and well-educated relatives, some memoir writers discovered that high social status offered little protection against rigid visitation rules. Hospitals justify early discharge by arguing that family members are knowledgeable enough to deliver competent medical care and are better qualified than health professionals to respond to patients' emotional needs. Inside many hospitals, however, staff viewed family members as ignorant and disruptive.[50]

The advice literature for caregivers urges them to play a major role in nursing homes. Pundits argue that because people remain in those facilities for the rest of their lives, it is essential that families monitor the quality of medical care and respond to emotional needs. People who have agonized over the decision to enroll relatives are often especially intent on remaining involved. But many quickly discover that they must tread lightly, fearful of antagonizing the staff members responsible for patients' overall well-being.

The Evolution of Hospice Care

Transforming the Role of Kin

Critics of the prevalence of high-intensity services at the end of life often point to hospices as a welcome alternative. They represent one form of palliative care, which views death as a natural event and seeks to enable people approaching mortality to live as fully and painlessly as possible. Unlike hospitals and nursing homes, hospices traditionally have assigned a major role to kin. Different generations of hospice leaders, however, have viewed that role very differently.

Hospices claim a distinguished lineage. The name comes from the way stations established by religious orders in the Middle Ages, where travelers to the holy lands were offered food and shelter. The US history, however, begins much more recently, with the 1963 visit by British doctor Cicely Saunders. Saunders lectured widely about her research on pain control for dying people and her vision for St. Christopher's in the Field, the hospice she soon established in England. Florence Schorske Wald, the dean of the Yale School of Nursing, was unable to attend the talk at Yale, but she arranged a special luncheon for Saunders, began a correspondence with her, and invited her to speak at the school in 1965.[1]

Born in 1917, Wald learned to value social justice as a child. "Both my parents were liberal in their thinking," she told an interviewer. "My father, for example, subscribed to *The Nation*, both my parents were registered in the Socialist Party and were champions of Norman Thomas." As an adult, Wald married an interest in psychiatry to her long-standing commitment to social reform. After graduating from the Yale School of Nursing in 1941, she worked first at the Visiting Nurse Service of New York and then at Babies Hospital, Columbia-Presbyterian, where she was introduced to Anna Freud's writings about the impact on children of separation from their parents. In 1955 she enrolled in an MS program in Mental Health Nursing at Yale and the following year joined the faculty of Rutgers University School of Nursing, teaching and working as an assistant to Hildegard E. Peplau. A follower of Harry Stack Sullivan, Peplau adapted his model of interpersonal relations to nursing practice. Peplau's influential theory emphasized the importance of the emotions of both nurses and patients and argued that the development of a relationship between them had therapeutic potential. In 1957 Wald returned to the Yale School of Nursing as a professor and became dean two years later. Eager to promote nursing research, Wald made contact with August B. Hollingshead, chair of the sociology department. We can assume she was especially interested in his *Social Class and Mental Illness: A Community Study* (1958), written with psychiatrist Fredrick C. Redlich. Wald also saw early drafts of *Sickness and Society* (1968), based on a study Hollingshead conducted at Yale–New Haven Hospital with pediatrician Raymond Duff.[2]

Wald recalled that Cicely Saunders "just opened the door to me." Saunders "solved the problem that both the faculty and the students were having in the hospital, seeing patients, particularly cancer patients, being treated with curative treatment, and where it was very obviously not curing the disease, but the suffering was so great. . . . They couldn't get the doctors to tell them what . . . the . . . outlook was for them, or to consider a variety of ways of treating the situation." In 1966 Saunders returned to Yale for six weeks, and the following year Wald took a sabbatical at St. Christopher's, now in operation in London. Soon after her return, she resigned her position as dean to devote herself to the establishment of the first US hospice.[3]

Saunders observed that dying people experienced "total pain" because their suffering had spiritual and emotional elements as well as physical ones. As her student, Wald assembled an interdisciplinary team to assist her in her endeavor. Edward Dobihal, chaplain at Yale–New Haven Hospital and a faculty member of the Yale Religious Studies Department, had studied psychotherapy. Morris Wessel, a pediatrician, had a strong interest in his patients' emotional well-being. The circle soon expanded to include Ira Goldenberg, an oncologist surgeon; Katherine Klaus, another nurse; and Robert Canny, a Catholic priest.[4]

Their first step was to conduct what they called "The Nurse's Study of the Terminally Ill Patient and His Family" (later "The Interdisciplinary Study of the Dying Patient and His Family"). Wald was familiar with the studies about hospital treatment of dying people that had appeared by the late 1960s. Four books—Barney G. Glaser and Anselm L. Strauss's *Aware-*

ness of Dying (1965) and *Time for Dying* (1968), Jeanne C. Quint's *The Nurse and the Dying Patient* (1967), and David Sudnow's *Passing On* (1967)—as well as a chapter in *Sickness and Society* signaled a rising discontent with hospital care for patients close to death. Together, they describe medical professionals who knew little about dying people, felt extremely uncomfortable interacting with them, concealed grim diagnoses and prognoses, and tried to concentrate on the patients most likely to recover. Wald and her colleagues added a critical dimension by focusing on the needs and wants of patients and family members not only in acute-care hospitals but also in chronic care facilities and at home.[5]

The inclusion of the family was significant. Wald later complained to an interviewer that one of the major problems with hospital care for dying people was that it "left the family out." Because terminal illness was traumatic for all members of the family, Wald argued, kin as well as patients needed supportive services. She frequently asserted that the family was the unit of care, a statement taken from the contemporary nursing literature. Her followers came to repeat it like a mantra.[6]

As the principal investigator, Wald devoted half her time to the study between 1969 and 1971. "One of the most important components of interpersonal theory," Hildegard E. Peplau wrote, "is its reliance on participant observation." Wald thus adhered to her mentor's theory when she assumed the role of participant observer, providing nursing services to twenty-two terminally ill hospital patients at Yale–New Haven Hospital. Although the study never was published, Yale University's Sterling Memorial Library has preserved the notes not only from Wald's interactions with patients and their relatives but also from the conferences she held with other health professionals and researchers to discuss the cases. Because Wald and her colleagues used those records as the basis for establishing a hospice, they help us understand how that group defined their relationship with both patients and kin.[7]

Rev. Edward Dobihal later noted that the goal was to listen to everybody, help people define their wants and needs, and explore how to fulfill them. But that project was more difficult than anticipated. Researchers did not always agree with patients and kin. The mother of one patient asserted that leeches should be applied. The wife of another wanted to bring her husband home so she could heal him with her cooking. Wald also quickly discovered that people did not always want to supply the information she sought. The first patient was a twenty-one-year-old woman who died of a liver disease soon after she entered the study. When Dobihal stated that she must have benefited from her short time with Wald, the patient's physician responded that the parents were happy their daughter had had extra care but that they had some "resentment" because they "thought their lives were being interfered with—their own personal lives—by questions." Another patient rebuffed Wald's inquiries by saying, "I have faced death, but I have not faced talking about it."[8]

Wald's extensive notes on one case indicate that she understood the need to refrain from delving too deeply into personal lives. Mrs. B., a woman dying of breast cancer, had three daughters, ages seven, fourteen, and nineteen. When Wald asked Mrs. B. how her children responded to her illness, she gave a "noncommittal answer," and "the conversation on this subject rather died out." Wald then commented, "I didn't feel comfortable in pushing it further." Because the oldest daughter was away at college and both the youngest daughter and the father rarely appeared, Wald had the most contact with Lisa, the fourteen-year-old. After meeting her the first time, Wald told Mrs. B. that she "certainly had a lovely girl, that she should be very proud of herself for bringing up such a nice girl." Because Mrs. B. offered little response, Wald wrote, "Again I felt I'd gone about as far in sharing this with her as I dared." Later, Wald admitted having made "a blunder" with Lisa. While discussing the need for another bed if the mother returned home, Wald had asked Lisa what such an event would mean to her. In retrospect, Wald realized, "it would have been much better had I not moved in on the feelings aspect of it." At other times, however, Wald assumed both mother and daughter were either shy or in denial when they gave vague answers to intimate questions or ignored them entirely.[9]

In addition, despite Dobihal's emphasis on the need to "listen" to everyone, Wald interpreted what she heard in terms of her own preconceptions about how patients should behave. According to a 1975 article that Wald coauthored with another nurse, "A nurse's hand, though full of skill, is not the same as the hand of a loved one to mop a brow, rub a back, or touch an arm." Moreover, "a family's active participation in care is . . . part of the separation process itself, which includes giving and receiving, coming together, and letting go." Wald thus reported approvingly when relatives helped hospital patients eat, wash, or go to the bathroom. Like Peplau, Wald also emphasized the benefits of expressing painful emotions. She thus en-

couraged both patients and family members—though often without success—to reveal their feelings of sadness, anger, and fear. When Mrs. B's
daughter Lisa responded to one of Wald's probing questions by saying that
she had done all her crying already, Wald told her she would have to do
some more.[10]

Ethnic stereotypes appear to have influenced Wald's interactions with
the family of Mr. R., an Italian immigrant who had suffered a bowel infarct
that had required extensive surgery. When conflicts erupted in the family,
Wald sided with the oldest son, Antonio, whom she considered the most
Americanized. He had been well educated and owned a hairdresser studio in
Westport, the wealthy suburb where she lived. The other children and their
parents were "what we call in Westport, you know, kind of 'greasers,' day
laborers, people who are interested in cars and [have] simple values." The
father "didn't have any outside interests, just family." His was a "very, very
restricted kind of life."[11]

Affluent individuals were another target of Wald's opprobrium. She asserted that one extremely wealthy patient could not deal with serious life
issues because she was spoiled and vain. In response to a suggestion that
the adolescent son of a dying woman live with his aunt, Wald argued that
the boy was extremely intelligent, creative, and industrious and therefore
could not fit into the aunt's "kind of country-club, superficial" household."[12]

If Wald's interest in patients and their relatives shaded easily into in-
trusiveness and moralizing, she and her colleagues also displayed enormous sensitivity to some of the issues family members confronted. One
question that frequently arose was where patients should spend the last
few weeks or months. Three options existed. Although administrators frequently asserted that they needed the beds of chronic care patients for
people with acute conditions, the study took place before the passage of
the Medicare prospective payment system for hospitals, encouraging early
discharge. Those facilities thus occasionally allowed people to remain for
lengthy periods. A few patients included in the study had been told they
could stay as long as they wanted. Alternatively, people could go to a nursing home or chronic disease hospital. Or they could return home, the usual
preference of families as well as patients.

But the last choice often entailed serious difficulties. Although Mrs. L.,
another woman with breast cancer, assumed she would be able to rely on
her mother when she left the hospital, her doctor reported that "her chest

wall malignancy [was] open and weeping and smelling and doing very poorly." Florence Wald and her colleagues thus doubted the mother could handle the dressings. Mrs. B. also had "a terribly big wound" that was "horrendous to see," according to Wald. Moreover, Lisa, the fourteen-year-old, often shared a bed with her mother. "If I recoil and really even the doctors recoil from that dressing," Wald continued, it was difficult to imagine Lisa sleeping near her mother. Moreover, because Mrs. B.'s mother was a difficult woman whom no one liked and her husband rarely was home, too much responsibility might fall on Lisa, who already was handling more than the group thought appropriate. The researchers also wanted to ensure that the seven-year-old had no opportunity to witness her mother's death, which doctors predicted would be bloody and painful.[13]

When members of Mr. R.'s family argued that they could care for him at home and demanded his return, his doctor pointed out that the man had an IV that needed to be changed often, "sometimes in the middle of the night." That procedure had become so difficult that the doctor "had to spend a half an hour with it the other night." Although Wald promised to visit the house regularly, she did not feel competent to handle the IV for a man with such poor veins. At his family's insistence, Mr. R. finally was sent home, but myriad problems arose. Unable to handle the IV's and feedings, the family became frantic and various members fell ill. The wife of one son left him, protesting that he spent too much time with his father. Mr. R's insurance coverage for home care was quickly exhausted. Forced to return to the hospital after a week, Mr. R. declared that he never wanted to impose such a strain on his family again.[14]

In yet another case, Wald and her colleagues could not understand why family members resisted bringing a patient home, until it became clear that they believed he could not walk. Because policymakers who endorse shifting care to the home frequently ignore the burdens bedridden patients impose on caregivers, the concerns Wald's team expressed are especially noteworthy. Although Wald occasionally idealized the care a loved one could provide, she and the rest of her group understood that the obligation easily could overwhelm.[15]

By 1971 they decided they had learned enough about dying people and their families to launch their own endeavor. Three years later, Hospice, Inc. (soon renamed the Connecticut Hospice), opened in New Haven, providing home care services to people who had a limited life expectancy. An inpatient facility opened in Branford in 1980. Sylvia Lack, the medical director, had worked at two London hospices and received Cicely Saunders's recommendation. Elisabeth Kübler-Ross was chairperson of the advisory council of the new facility and Saunders a consultant. Wald's tenure, however, was brief. The Board of Directors repeatedly heard complaints that she tried to micromanage the program she had founded, and in 1975 she was asked to resign.[16]

Nevertheless, Wald remained actively involved in the hospice movement, traveling frequently throughout the country, promoting hospices as a compassionate alternative to high-tech hospital care for dying people. By the early 1980s, hundreds of other hospices were in existence. Most were small, grassroots efforts that differed widely from one another. Although a newly established National Hospice Organization formulated a set of standards in 1978, few programs adhered to them.[17]

We can explain the eager embrace of the hospice idea in several ways. Elisabeth Kübler-Ross's *On Death and Dying* appeared in 1969, publicizing longstanding critiques of American care for dying people, which hospices sought to address. As we have seen, a growing number of health professionals had begun to question medical secrecy by the late 1960s. Although acknowledging that some individuals did not want to know the full details of their conditions, hospice leaders placed a premium on physician honesty, arguing that dying people could prepare for death only if they knew when it was imminent.[18]

Hospices also tried to counter the social isolation of people near the end of life, another issue Kübler-Ross highlighted. Hospice advocates condemned hospital regulations that disrupted intimate ties just when the need for them was greatest. At the forty-four-bed inpatient facility Hospice, Inc., established in 1978, all patient rooms were large enough to accommodate several family members at one time. Despite Florence Wald's sensitivity to the needs of family caregivers, most hospices extolled the value of home care. "The home is the natural place to die," declared a pamphlet distributed by Hospice, Inc. "Protected from institutional encroachments upon their dignity, and thereby able to maintain individuality, the dying can avoid the isolation and anonymity that is too often their lot."[19]

Another reason the hospice movement expanded so rapidly is that it arose during a period of widespread social reform. Florence Wald and her colleagues participated actively in the social movements of the 1960s and early 1970s. "During the course of our original research," Wald later remarked, "we were as apt to meet at vigils for peace, meetings in the black ghettoes of New Haven on behalf of their civil rights as we were in corridors, clinics, and meeting rooms of the medical center." She commented that reform also reached medicine. Hospices may have seemed especially appealing because they incorporated the ideas of diverse health care reform movements. The holistic health movement demanded that patients be viewed as whole human beings, not simply the sum of their symptoms. The women's health movement criticized physician secrecy and the technological focus of modern medicine; a branch, the natural childbirth movement, complained about the medicalization of pivotal life events. Wald pointed to the resemblance between the natural childbirth movement and the hospice movement, noting that both received support from women's health activists in the 1970s.[20]

And various groups challenged the established order by organizing what were called "counterinstitutions," which represented alternatives to established ones. For example, free schools, food cooperatives, and alternative newspapers sought to curtail the sovereignty of experts by sharing skills and rotating tasks. Hospices resembled those institutions in various ways. Hospices, of course, could not afford to disregard all professional competence. The judgment and knowledge of physicians were essential for the alleviation of pain and the determination of when death was imminent. Nevertheless, hospice advocates insisted that human life was more than "a breathing lung and beating heart" and that dying people had spiritual, social, and emotional needs, not just physical problems. Many programs thus tried to regard physicians as just one group among a variety of equal members of an interdisciplinary team.[21]

Hospices also shared with other counterinstitutions the goal of increasing acceptance of nature. The technological, curative focus of modern medicine, hospice proponents claimed, had distorted the process of death. They attributed much of the agony of dying people to futile treatments and sought to dispense with heroic, life-sustaining therapies. Like other counterinstitutions, hospices also challenged the bureaucratization of established social services. "The primary message that must be conveyed to the dying patient," one hospice champion asserted, "is that he is unique and that his needs are special and will be met in an individual way." Disregarding conventional criteria of productivity, many hospices allowed each patient visit to take as long as necessary. Regimentation also was avoided in the delivery of care. Hospices exhibited respect for individual differences by allowing patients to set their own schedules, wear their own clothes, and keep their own possessions; inpatient facilities had no restrictions on visiting hours.[22]

Another similarity between hospices and the counterinstitutions of the late 1960s and early 1970s was an initial indifference to finances. That cavalier attitude stemmed partly from a belief that a crass concern with money was antithetical to the hospice mission. To commodify the work of caring would be to diminish its significance. Moreover, hospice leaders were aware that all money comes with strings attached. Believing that traditional third-party payers had distorted the health care system, some of the first hospices provided services free of charge. Others relied exclusively on public and private grants and individual donations.

One way hospices saved money was by emphasizing home care. A 1975 fund-raising appeal by Hospice, Inc., noted that the average cost of hospital care for patients with advanced cancer was $21,718; for nearly one-third of such patients, the cost was between $25,000 and $50,000. By providing most of their services outside institutions, hospices greatly reduced that enormous expense. Hospices also cut costs by relying on a cadre of volunteers. For many hospice leaders, the recruitment of volunteers was not just a matter of expedience. Hospice advocates asserted that the absence of remuneration demonstrated dedication and commitment. Because volunteers reaped no extrinsic rewards, their work truly could be considered a labor of love. Like other counterinstitutions, hospices also tried to remain apart from mainstream institutions. The founders wanted to start afresh, unencumbered by the practices, traditions, and regulations of the health care system. As a result, the great majority of hospices began as independent agencies.[23]

But complete separation was as impossible for hospices as it was for other counterinstitutions. Forced to rely on the traditional health care system for resources, political acceptance, and personnel, hospices gradually accommodated themselves to the established order and lost much of their distinctiveness. Despite the desire for autonomy, a growing number of hospice programs were housed in hospitals or home health agencies. All hospices found it necessary to strive for credibility in the medical community, because they depended on hospital discharge planners and private physicians for referrals and continued to work closely with attending physicians after patients' admission. Some hospices sought legitimacy by appointing physicians as directors of the interdisciplinary teams.

In addition, the majority of hospices discovered that they could not continue to rely exclusively on grants and thus sought reimbursement from public and private insurance programs. Third-party reimbursement required more formalized and sophisticated management structures. Nursing staffs were instructed to document their services more scrupulously than before, to place greater emphasis on efficiency, and, occasionally, to adhere to rigid standards of productivity. Most hospices also hired separate administrative staff responsible for record-keeping and finances. Changes in the composition of boards of trustees occasionally mirrored those other trends. Bank officers, financial managers, and lawyers gradually replaced clergy, health care providers, and community representatives.[24]

More than any other event, the addition of hospice as a covered Medicare benefit in the Tax, Equity, and Fiscal Responsibility Act (TEFRA) moved hospices into the mainstream. Passed in August 1982, the legislation was signed by President Ronald Reagan the following month. The early 1980s was a period of economic retrenchment. As a result, the financial considerations that early hospice leaders had viewed with disdain preoccupied many proponents of that legislation. Most observers agree that Congress endorsed the Medicare hospice benefit to contain health care costs. Alarmed by the amount of government money spent on caring for elderly people in their final months of life, legislators were eager to find a way to reduce that expense. Growing popular support for hospice ideals undoubtedly facilitated the passage of the benefit, but that outcome was ensured by a report of the Congressional Budget Office, concluding that the government could save as much as $1,120 for each Medicare beneficiary who enrolled in hospice. A sunset clause limited the benefit to a three-year period; renewal would depend on a report on the program's cost-effectiveness. (Two other components of TEFRA—increasing the use of health maintenance organizations and instituting a prospective payment system—also were promoted as ways to save money.)[25]

Legislators set the hospice payment cap at 75 percent of the average cost of caring for Medicare beneficiaries in hospitals in the last six months of life, subsequently reducing it to 40 percent—far too low, many hospice leaders argued, to enable them to provide high-quality services. The savings were to come primarily from the continued reliance on unpaid relatives. Robert Dole, who introduced the hospice provision in the Senate, later asserted that its passage "was possible because many believe, as I do, that it is less costly to care for a patient at home, foregoing expensive hospital treatment." To ensure that care shifted from hospitals to the home, the legislation limited the number of inpatient days a hospice could provide to 20 percent of the total patient days. Although Wald and her colleagues had stressed the cost-effectiveness of hospice care, they had tried to attend to the myriad problems family caregivers faced when death was imminent, albeit with varying amounts of success. An anthropologist who studied family members helping people die at home during the late 1980s, shortly after the passage of TEFRA, found that although the work could be extremely rewarding, it also made enormous physical and emotional demands: "Common actions and activities that people take for granted can become overwhelming problems and ordeals for patient and caregiver. Eating, sleeping, taking a pill, drinking a glass of water, elimination, taking a bath, keeping the patient clean, turned and free from bedsores, going outside—all represent major undertakings for both." Common procedures caregivers were expected to perform included suctioning, catheterization, disimpaction of bowels, the administration of enemas, and injections. Nevertheless, the burdens of caring for dying patients at home received little attention in congressional hearings on the Medicare provision. To many advocates of the hospice benefit, relatives appear to have represented primarily a cheap form of labor.[26]

The legislation also created a bureaucratic structure, imposing uniformity and rigid rules on programs that had prided themselves on innovation and diversity. To receive reimbursement under the Medicare benefit, programs had to employ certain types of staff, admit certain types of patients, and provide a specific set of services.

TEFRA accelerated the transformation of a movement into an industry. Although many hospice leaders complained that the cap was grossly inadequate, the infusion of government funding was sufficiently large to attract investors. Shortly after the enactment of TEFRA, a former president of the National Hospice Organization announced plans to open a chain of for-profit hospices. Since then, the number of for-profit institutions has steadily grown. By 2012 more than fifty-five hundred hospices were in existence, serving 1.5 million to 1.6 million people. More than half of the programs were for-profit entities, many attached to national chains.[27]

Enrollment figures, however, do not tell the whole story. More than one-third of patients enter hospices within seven days of death, too late, many commentators believe, to take advantage of the full range of services. Observers commonly explain late admissions by pointing to the failure of doctors to clearly communicate poor prognoses and the refusal of both patients and families to abandon hope of cure.[28]

Observers attribute other problems to the business ethos that increasingly has replaced the idealism of the early movement. Many hospices, for example, reject patients who require chemotherapy and radiation. That policy stems in part from history: throughout the 1970s and 1980s, those therapies were administered only when they offered some promise of cure. But the line between curative and palliative treatments increasingly has faded; physicians now use chemotherapy and radiation to improve the quality of life of terminally ill patients. The primary disadvantage of the treatments now, many commentators charge, is their expense. Most hospices limit admission to patients who have primary caregivers at home, another policy that reflects both the original hospice mission and the current emphasis on cost containment. In addition, hospices increasingly discharge patients before death. In some cases, the patients may have improved or decided to resume curative treatment. In others, however, the motive is to avoid paying for costly care. "When you have a live discharge rate that is as high as 30 percent, you have to wonder whether a hospice program is living up to the vision and morality of the founders," one researcher commented, adding that "some of the new hospice providers may . . . be more concerned with profit margins than compassionate care." For-profit hospices have more restrictive enrollment policies and higher discharge rates than non-profit ones.[29]

A growing number of family memoirs published after the early 1980s discussed hospices. In some cases, the services were enlisted at the very end. We recall that Amanda Bennett and her husband Terrence Foley pursued an extremely aggressive course of treatment, searching for new medications even after any hope for recovery had faded. When doctors told Bennett that the end was imminent, she refused to consider hospice care. Eventually, however, she reconsidered. Because the hospital had a hospice program that could be administered in the room Foley occupied, his bed was converted from hospital to hospice. Bennett described what happened next: "The hospital staff takes away the machines and the monitors. They remove the oxygen tubes. They silence the steady click of the heart monitor. The green wiggly lines above his head go dark. The oncologists and radiologist and lab technicians disappear. Another group of people—hospice nurses, social workers, chaplains, and counselors—appear to help Terrence, me, and the children." But hospice represented less a different form of care than the prelude to death. Three days later Foley was gone.[30]

In other cases, patients remained in hospice care for a longer period of time. In accord with their desire to keep disturbing information from their dying relatives, some family members obtained hospice services without informing the patients. John Thorndike recalled that his father realized "something strange was going on" when a new nurse arrived at the house, but he did not understand she was from a hospice. "He knows what Hospice is," Thorndike explained, "and wouldn't want anything to do with it, wouldn't want to hear the word spoken." Valerie Seiling Jacobs placed her father in an inpatient hospice. "Not that I ever used that word in from of him," she wrote. "To have used the *H* word would have been to admit defeat and, more important, to abandon hope." The woman from the facility who came to his hospital room to conduct an intake interview had a lanyard with the word *Hospice* displayed in bold letters. "Do you have to wear that?" Jacobs asked. "It's just that I haven't told him where he's going." She then watched as the woman "slowly flipped the badge over, so that only the plain white backing was visible."[31]

A few memoirs described hospices fulfilling their goal of delivering holistic care. We saw in chapter 1 that a high proportion of memoir writers criticized doctors who attended only to the disease, not the person. By contrast, many of the hospice workers described in the narratives were successful in addressing patients' psychological and spiritual preoccupations as well as their physical pain and suffering. Sara Evans, for example, wrote that "Solace" was "a good name" for the "wonderful facility" where her mother spent her final days. "From the moment she arrived she was enfolded in a community of caregivers whose sole purpose [was] comfort on every level—physical, emotional, spiritual." Katy Butler recalled that when her father was dying, "the hospice nurses, practiced at filling the spiritual vacuums of contemporary life, would minister to us unobtrusively, the way priests and family members once did. I was grateful." Shortly before the death of Butler's mother the following year, another hospice worker helped to heal a bitter conflict. After the mother and her son Michael had "a classic, familiar fight," initiated by the mother's attempt to limit how much he ate, he demanded that Katy buy him a plane ticket home. She agreed but suggested he wait a few hours. "With help from a hospice social worker conducting shuttle diplomacy, he and my mother began talking again, this time in earnest and with care. He spoke to her for hours about the pain of their intense, difficult relationship, stretching back to his childhood." His mother was able to "listen and acknowledge."[32]

A few writers also described hospice staff caring with unusual warmth and attentiveness. Recalling the hospice nurse he had seen "adjusting Mom's pillow or dabbing the corners of her eyes or giving her gentle sips of water," Will Schwalbe commented, "It was an extraordinary sight—a stranger tending to our mother with infinite care." John Thorndike remembered one of the aides who cared for his father as "dark-eyed, calm and always beautifully dressed. . . . She says a few soft sentences to my father and wins him over with her calm and reserve."[33]

Many more writers expressed gratitude for the practical assistance they received. Diane Rubin had been the primary caregiver for her mother for more than two years. "Perhaps they seem like trivial things," Diane wrote, "some phone calls and some simple arrangements. But to us—to *me* especially—it was a blessing to have someone else in charge." After talking for two hours with the hospice admissions nurse, Stan Mack "felt the weight of desperation begin to lift." When the nurse said that "hospice would arrange things with the health insurance carrier and supply medications, I thought, no more fighting with billing, no more last-minute drugstore runs, no more confusion about dosage adjustments and equipment . . . thank you, thank you." Hospices also furnished medical equipment and hospital beds. The bed delivered by a local hospice enabled Laurie Foos's father to die at home in a "room with the day bed and eyelet pillows, my mother's lacy white curtains." And hospice staff provided invaluable instruction. Families learned how to lift bedridden patients, recognize the signs of active dying, and administer pain medication.[34]

But many writers complained that the amount of help hospices offered was seriously inadequate. "Even the most astute caregiver," Kathryn Temple wrote, "might have difficulty getting past the hospice promotional literature to discover just what the limits of the promised 'care' might be." It is perhaps significant that the family members who were most positive about hospice care tended either to have placed patients in hospice facilities or to have been able to pay for additional services at home. Hillary Johnson, by contrast, wrote that as her mother "deteriorated, her care became exponentially complicated and demanding. A hospice nurse would visit each day, but for the remaining twenty-three hours, we were on our own."[35]

Although some writers praised the emotional care hospice staff dispensed, others deprecated it. "In our meeting with the hospice psychiatrist and hospice social worker," Diane Rubin wrote, "we made it clear we didn't wish to share our feelings and frustrations anymore. What was the point?" Mark Doty does not appear to have solicited hospice services, but the nurse who arrived at his house clearly had absorbed the hospice message about the importance of rendering psychological counsel. We saw that, like the parents of the first patient Florence Wald interviewed for the Nurse's Study, Doty resented the interference in his personal life. "Of all the things that have annoyed and troubled me about the medical people Wally and I dealt with," he later wrote, "perhaps what I hated most was the seemingly endemic practice of assuming that patients *needed* counseling and that whoever happened to be around was the one to do it."[36]

Kathryn Temple challenged the hospice commitment to home care: "Perhaps the most difficult issue our family faced involved the continual pressure to care for my husband at home." Her situation was "particularly unsuited to in-home hospice care. No local family members, my only friends all from two-career families with children and plenty of problems of their own, my husband, a patient who needed twenty-four-hour care, had unpredictable bleeding and an active case of hepatitis B." Moreover, as in the case of Mr. R. (the Italian father Florence Wald discussed in 1969), Temple had a young daughter at home, and doctors warned the death would not be easy. One hospital nurse who worked part time at a local hospice angrily asked why Temple did not bring her husband home so her daughter could see him. "Did I really need to explain," Temple asked, "that I had stopped bringing my daughter to visit only after my husband's symptoms had become so disturbing that even adult visitors were having nightmares?"[37]

Finally, writers complained about the problems they believed stemmed from bureaucratic rigidity. Jean Levitan, a professor of public health at William Paterson University of New Jersey, learned from her uncle about the care her aunt received. "Rather than truly getting the palliative care

that is supposedly a staple of hospice," Levitan reported, "she was neglected, and both she and my uncle felt abandoned by a system that would
only respond as long as all the paperwork was correct ensuring proper payment once submitted. Responses to their requests for help seemed to be
constantly framed within the need for medical personnel to first get the
proper authorizations; attending to her pain was secondary."[38]

Eligibility criteria excluded certain patients. For many years, hospices
limited enrollment to people with cancer, because that disease tended to
follow a predictable trajectory. Meryl Comer explained what happened the
three times a doctor referred her husband Harvey, who had Alzheimer's
disease, to hospice care. Each time his health stabilized, he was "dropped
from the list." Other writers criticized regulations preventing hospice staff
from discussing physician-assisted suicide with patients. And Richard
Lischer charged that adherence to a rule that hospice patients not receive
curative treatment added to his son Adam's agony the day before he died.
When OxyContin failed to alleviate Adam's terrible pain, the oncologist
decided he should be admitted to the hospital. While he waited for an
available room, the hospice dispatched a nurse with a more powerful medication. "In the crisis hour, when things couldn't get worse," the father later
wrote, "they somehow did. When the hospice nurse was informed that
we were trying to have Adam admitted to the hospital, she turned around
and refused to come to the house. Jenny [Adam's wife] tried to explain—I
could hear her pleading—that his hospitalization would have nothing to
do with treatment, only the palliation of pain, but to no avail."[39]

Conclusion

Florence Wald argued more than forty years ago that the physical
and emotional demands of caring for dying people at home become too burdensome. Since then, the number of home deaths has increased, at least in
part as a result of the movement she helped to launch. Partly for financial
reasons, most early hospices emphasized home care. The passage of the
1983 Medicare hospice benefit rested not only on the argument that hospices offered a superior form of care but also on the contention that they
saved money by relying on the free labor of families. Today there is re-
newed pressure to shift more deaths out of institutions. Advocates argue
that most people want to die at home but just one-third do so, that hospitals often provide futile treatments at the end of life, and that home care is

far less expensive than care in either nursing homes or hospitals. But the memoirs remind us of the need to focus on the needs of kin, not just on those of patients.[40]

It is easy to wax nostalgic about the nineteenth century, when family and friends sat by dying people, offering comfort, administering medications, and watching for dangerous symptoms. But the reality of nineteenth-century deaths was often very different from our idealized image of it. And care for dying people at home is much more difficult today than it was in the past, largely because the patients are sicker and caregiving responsibilities more complex. Designed as cost-containment mechanisms, hospices cannot compensate for all the work institutions provide. In most cases, a hospice nurse visits one hour each day. Family members can call for advice at other times as well. Most of the time, however, they are completely on their own. Originally designed as a way to treat the entire family as a unit of care, hospices increasingly have relied on kin as a cheap form of labor.

Conclusion

Dying in America, a 2014 Institute of Medicine report, called attention to the increasingly common route to the end of life: "For most people, death does not come suddenly. Instead, dying is an inevitable result of one or more diseases that must be managed carefully and compassionately over weeks, months, or even years, through many ups and down." Nevertheless, like most contemporary observers, the report focused almost exclusively on the drama surrounding the very last phase of life. The family memoirs explored in this book highlight the need to redirect attention to the entire course of life-threatening chronic disease.[1]

Virtually all memoirists vividly recalled the moment of diagnosis, which shattered the world they had known. As the era of medical paternalism gradually receded, doctors became more willing to name the disease. But many writers had difficulty learning what to expect. Another common complaint was that doctors transmitted grim diagnoses and prognoses impersonally and occasionally even brutally, ignoring the emotional impact of the news they delivered. The doctor who revealed that leukemia had struck Gordon Livingston's six-year-old son spoke openly about the gravity of the boy's condition, but Livingston remained dissatisfied. He wanted some indication that the doctor understood that the family would be changed forever.

When conventional medicine could not halt the progress of disease, many individuals pinned their hopes on experimental treatments. Long after the media began to report examples of gross abuse of human subjects, most memoirists remained convinced that the interests of researchers and patients coincided. Although Doris Lund's son Eric underwent extremely brutal experimental therapies, Doris praised his doctors for refusing to surrender. She expressed reservation about his treatment only at the very end of his life, when he was unconscious and his doctor recommended a medication that could not possibly work. Gerda Lerner's 1978 memoir, *A*

Death of One's Own, was unusual in questioning the goal of medical research, but even she eventually applauded the enterprise. Beginning in the 1980s, people with AIDS and later those confronting other diseases distanced themselves from medical authority. Nevertheless, skepticism of individual practitioners did not necessarily disabuse people of the belief that entry into the next clinical trial could produce a remission or a cure. Even as death approached, Amanda Bennett and Susan Sontag refused to relinquish the hope that one more innovative treatment might reverse the disease trajectory.

At some point, most patients and family members realized that medicine could not avert death. Some placed their faith in mind-body practices. Others turned to religion for the miracle cure medicine had failed to deliver. And several found in religion a way to understand the anguish health care providers did not address. As theologian Richard Lischer wrote, "Suffering, with its many depths and its mysterious interplay of body and spirit, is beyond the scope of pain and therefore beyond the competence of most medical practitioners." Lischer's dying son Adam continued treatment while he intensified his own religious devotion, but other patients suspended all therapy when they entered what two memoir writers called "a sacred time."

The memoirists repeatedly complained that while they struggled to accept the inevitability of human finitude, other people in their lives adamantly denied it. Friends disappeared, doctors prevaricated, and nurses hid behind falsely cheerful demeanors. But it was one thing to criticize the culture of denial and quite another to maintain that acceptance was essential to a good death, an argument most closely identified with Elisabeth Kübler-Ross. Having tried unsuccessfully to shape relatives' emotions, several writers concluded that dying individuals must find their own way to approach the end. Kathryn Temple had initially believed that her husband needed to understand his dismal prognosis so that he could participate in treatment decisions and make the best use of his remaining time. When he resisted Temple's attempts to tell him the truth, however, she realized his choice demanded respect. As a poet, Mark Doty was better able than many family members to tolerate ambiguity and uncertainty, and he bitterly resented the nurse who tried to structure his lover's feelings. When Doty knew death was imminent, he still used denial to get through the day.

Several memoir authors joined that vast army of family caregivers who provide the great bulk of long-term care in America. The intense emotional involvement of many writers in that activity suggests that they did not view themselves solely as filling gaps in the health care system. Nevertheless, some people felt compelled to provide far more care than they wanted. Although the memoirists were relatively affluent, few could afford home health aides for extended periods, and many recoiled from the thought of putting their relatives in nursing homes. More than a quarter century after the Nursing Home Reform Act of 1987, study after study relentlessly reports substandard conditions. Patients funded by Medicaid tend to receive the worst care. Although none of the memoir writers had to rely on Medicaid at the time of initial placement, many responded with horror to the facilities they investigated. Thus, despite the serious, often calamitous, costs that caregiving imposed on their own lives, some authors kept relatives home long after professionals recommended they leave.

The memoirs also reveal that the rise of a self-help industry for caregivers represents an inadequate response to the problems they encounter. To be sure, some advice helped family members develop coping capacities. Those caring for people with dementia were especially likely to feel they were negotiating new turf with few familiar signposts to guide them. Several believed that they could more easily tolerate troubling and even frightening actions if they understood the genesis of those behaviors and learned techniques for dealing with them. But other memoirists complained that the advice they received had limited value. Some did not want to view their relatives through the lens of disease. And some contended that the literature focused primarily on their attitudes while ignoring the economic realities of their lives. A freelance writer caring for a mother with dementia, Eleanor Cooney had too much money to qualify for public services and too little to pay for private care. As a result, she wrote, her level of stress was especially high.

Regardless of whether they delivered care at home or in institutions, memoir writers tried to treat their relatives as singular and irreplaceable human beings. Disease and institutional regulations, however, retarded their efforts. Some believed dementia had ravaged a relative's personhood. And despite the success of some campaigns to open ICUs to families and allow them to witness resuscitation efforts, many memoirists blamed hospitals and nursing homes for restricting their presence and disregarding their input. The evidence suggests that nurses and doctors accord special consideration to privileged groups, but a few authors complained about being banished at the moment of death. High social status also did not guarantee that the authors could obtain what they considered good care for their relatives. The celebrated sportscaster Frank Deford had no power to alter the humiliating way doctors in a major academic medical center treated his dying daughter. Others, although shocked by the dismal treatment their parents received in nursing homes, tried to complain as little as possible.

When death approached, several authors enrolled their relatives in hospices. Those programs have helped to counter the growing focus on aggressive, often futile, therapy at the end of life by delivering palliative care. Following Cicely Saunders's injunction to concentrate on the "total pain" of dying people, hospices historically have prided themselves on providing not only relief from physical symptoms but also the emotional and spiritual support many memoir writers found lacking elsewhere in the health care system. But not all professionals are able to bestow compassionate care, and not all patients and family members want to receive it. Some writers appreciated the unusual warmth of hospice staff and the personal interest they displayed. Others, however, complained about insensitive comments and intrusion into private affairs. An equally serious criticism was that hospices failed to provide adequate practical and medical assistance. Florence Wald, the founder of the first US hospice, emphasized the myriad difficulties many families encountered in caring for dying people at home. But because many policymakers have viewed hospices primarily as a way to save money, the programs have accelerated the movement of death out of nursing homes and hospitals without providing the services those institutions deliver. Hillary Johnson recalled that as her mother approached death, her care became far more complex and demanding. Like most hospices, the one in which Johnson's mother was enrolled sent a visiting nurse just one hour each day. For the rest of the time, the family had to fend for itself.

Coming on the heels of the mischaracterization of conversations about end-of-life wishes as death panels during the debate about the Affordable Care Act, the Institute of Medicine's report *Dying in America* repeatedly stressed the need for advance care planning, including a medical power of attorney and a living will stating treatment preferences. Those directives are crucial because many people facing imminent death are incapable of making decisions about "do not resuscitate" orders and life-prolonging technologies. But preoccupation with those issues has diverted attention from the many other, equally consequential questions that arise throughout a long illness.[2]

Among the dilemmas memoir writers faced are these: How much negative information should they disclose to adult relatives? To children? When should the adult daughter of a mother with dementia begin to consider nursing home placement? How should the daughter balance her own need for relief from caregiving with the mother's fervent desire to remain at home? How should a father choose between two possible treatments for his young son with leukemia? Should the boy have chemotherapy alone, with a 40 percent chance of extending life, or a bone marrow transplant, which is much more dangerous and brutal but has a 70 percent probability of success? Should parents give permission for a second brain surgery for their eighteen-year-old son after the first one has altered him almost beyond recognition? How could a mother determine whether her son's seizures were new neurological symptoms of AIDS or side effects of his new medication? When should she insist he call the doctor? And above all, how can anyone come to terms with the impending loss of a child? To people who had confronted those questions, debates about "do not resuscitate" orders, feeding tubes, and respirators could seem relatively insignificant.

Dying today is often an extremely protracted process, not only because new technologies can extend a person's final days or weeks, but even more because many people live for years with one or more terminal conditions. Nevertheless, we continue to ignore the long course of dying, emphasizing instead the brief period when death is imminent. The family memoirs we have explored underline the urgency of turning our attention to a host of other critical issues, including the miserable quality of nursing home care, the restrictive visitation regulations imposed by intensive care units, the lack of emotional and spiritual support for people confronting death, the business concerns that increasingly influence hospice services, the secrecy that continues to surround both prognoses and the goals of clinical trials, and the widespread belief that the care of people suffering from life-threatening illness is primarily a family, not a social, responsibility.

Acknowledgments

Once again I thank my history writing group, Carla Bittel, Janet Farrell Brodie, Lisa Cody, Sharla Fett, Terri Snyder, and Alice Wexler, for their trenchant comments, gourmet meals, and fun. Rick Abel, Marcia Meldrum, Andrea Sankar, Susan Smith, and Jacqueline Wolf also read parts of the manuscript and provided insightful suggestions.

Like Jacqueline Wehmueller's many other authors, I have relied heavily on her wisdom and encouragement. She expressed interest in the project from the beginning, made invaluable suggestions, and commented on draft after draft. Patricia D'Antonio read the manuscript for the press; I followed her recommendations almost to the letter. Lois Crum provided excellent copyediting.

Because my family and friends begged me to find a more cheerful topic this time, I especially appreciate their love and support even as I disobeyed their wishes.

Notes

Introduction

1. Joanne Lynn, *Sick to Death and Not Going to Take It Anymore!* (Berkeley: University of California Press, 2004), p. 139; Helen Schulman, "My Father the Garbage Head," in *An Uncertain Inheritance: Writers on Caring for Family,* ed. Nell Casey (New York: Harper, 2007), p. 1.

2. Carl E. Schneider, *The Practice of Autonomy: Patients, Doctors, and Medical Decisions* (New York: Oxford University Press, 1998), p. 1; David J. Rothman, *Strangers at the Bedside: A History of How Law and Bioethics Transformed Medical Decision Making* (New Brunswick, NJ: Aldine Transaction, 2011; first published 1991), p. 1.

3. Virginia Held, introduction to *Justice and Care: Essential Readings in Feminist Ethics,* ed. Virginia Held (Boulder: Westview Press, 1995), p. 1.

4. Institute of Medicine, *Improving Quality and Honoring Individual Preferences near the End of Life* (Washington, DC: National Academies Press, 2014), p. S-9; Tamar Lewin, "Nancy Cruzan Dies, Outlived by a Debate over the Right to Die," *New York Times,* December 27, 1990. Both of the memoirs that mentioned a struggle over letting a person die were published in 1991, shortly after the US Supreme Court ruled in the Nancy Cruzan case, which had sparked a bitter public debate about the right to die. One memoir was by a journalist who had focused extensively on end-of-life issues. The second author was Philip Roth, who previously had faced far more agonizing decisions in the course of his father's illness. Andrew H. Malcolm, *Someday: The Story of a Mother and Her Son* (New York: Alfred A. Knopf, 1991); Philip Roth, *Patrimony* (New York: Random House, 1991).

5. Bruce C. Vladeck, *Unloving Care: The Nursing Home Tragedy* (New York: Basic Books, 1983); O. G. Brim, H. E. Freeman, S. Levine, and N. A. Scotch, *The Dying Patient* (New York: Russell Sage Foundation, 1970); Rosemary Stevens, *In Sickness and in Wealth: American Hospitals in the Twentieth Century* (New York: Basic Books, 1989), p. 231; Rick Mayes, "The Origins, Development, and Passage of Medicare's Revolutionary Prospective Payment System," *Journal of the History of Medicine and Allied Sciences* 62, no. 1 (2007): 21–55; Institute of Medicine, *Dying in America: Improving Quality and Honoring Individual Preferences near the End of Life* (Washington, DC: National Academies Press, 2014), pp. 5–25; N. R. Kleinfield, "The Lonely Death of George Bell," *New York Times,* October 18, 2015.

6. Julie Fairman and Joan Lynaugh, *Critical Care Nursing: A History* (Philadelphia: University of Pennsylvania Press, 1998).

7. Joy Buck, "Reweaving a Tapestry of Care: Religion, Nursing, and the Meaning of Hospice, 1945–1978," *Nursing History Review* 15 (2007): 133.

8. Elliot G. Mishler, *The Discourse of Medicine: Dialectics of Medical Interviews* (Norwood, NJ: Ablex, 1984); Roy Porter, "The Patient's View," *Theory and Society* 14 (1985): 192; Arthur Kleinman, *The Illness Narratives: Suffering, Healing and the Human Condition* (New York: Basic Books, 1988). See also Cheryl Mattingly and Linda Garro, eds., *Narrative and Social Construction of Illness and Healing* (Berkeley: University of California Press, 2000); Rita Charon, *Narrative Medicine: Honoring the Stories of Illness* (New York: Oxford University Press, 2006); Peter D. Kramer, "Why Doctors Need Stories," *New York Times*, October 18, 2014.

9. Flurin Condrau, "The Patient's View Meets the Clinical Gaze," *Social History of Medicine* 20, no 3 (2007): 525–40; Catriona Stoljar and Natalie Mackenzie, eds., *Relational Autonomy* (New York: Oxford University Press, 2000).

10. Andrew J. Cherlin, *The Marriage-Go-Round: The State of Marriage and the Family in America Today* (New York: Random House, 2009).

11. Emily K. Abel, *Hearts of Wisdom: American Women Caring for Kin, 1840–1965* (Cambridge, MA: Harvard University Press, 2000).

12. Samuel J. Crumbine, *Frontier Doctor: The Autobiography of a Pioneer on the Frontier of Public Health* (Philadelphia: Dorrance, 1948), p. 153; George Rosen, *The Structure of American Medical Practice, 1875–1941* (Philadelphia: University of Pennsylvania Press, 1983); William Allen Pusey, *A Doctor of the 1870s and 80s* (Springfield, IL: Charles C. Thomas, 1932), p. 94.

13. Kenneth M. Ludmerer, *Time to Heal: American Medical Education from the Turn of the Century to the Era of Managed Care* (New York: Oxford University Press), p. 109; Abel, *Hearts of Wisdom*.

14. Carol Levine and Connie Zuckerman, "Hands On / Hands Off: Why Health Care Professionals Depend on Families but Keep Them at Arm's length," *Journal of Law, Medicine, and Ethics* 28 (2000): 7.

15. Condrau, "Patient's View"; Lars-Christer Hydén, "Illness and Narratives," *Sociology of Health and Illness* 19, no. 1 (1997): 48–69.

16. G. Thomas Couser, *Recovering Bodies: Illness, Disability, and Life Writing* (Madison: University of Wisconsin Press, 1997); Schneider, *Practice of Autonomy;* Marcia Friedman, *The Story of Josh* (New York: Ballantine Books, 1974), p. 136. A study published in 2009 found that the cost of medical services accounted for nearly half of all bankruptcies in the United States. See David U. Himmelstein, Deborah Thorne, Elizabeth Warren, and Steffie Woolhandler, "Medical Bankruptcy in the United States, 2007: Results of a National Study," *American Journal of Medicine* 122, no. 8 (August 2009): 741–46.

17. Ben Yagoda, *Memoir: A History* (New York: Riverhead Books, 2009), p. 7; Daniel Mendelsohn, "But Enough about Me: What Does the Popularity of Memoirs Tell Us about Ourselves?," *New Yorker*, January 25, 2010.

18. Neil Genzlinger, "The Problem with Memoirs," *New York Times Book Review*, January 30, 2011. See William Grimes, "We All Have a Life: Must We All Write about It?," *New York Times*, March 25, 2005; Michiko Kakutani, "Woe Is Me: Rewards and Perils of Memoirs," *New York Times Book Review*, October 21, 1997; Catherine Sailent, "Gone with the Wind? No Way," *Los Angeles Times*, October 15, 2005; Judith Shulevitz, "My True Story," review of *Memoir: A History*, by Ben Yagoda, *New York Times*, November 11, 2009;

Jonathan Yardley, review of *Memoir: A History,* by Ben Yagoda, *Washington Post,* November 29, 2009; William Zinsser, "The Right to Write," *American Scholar,* February 18, 2011.

19. See Catherine Kohler Riessman, *Narrative Methods for the Human Sciences* (Los Angeles: Sage, 2008), p. 9; Paula Fass, "The Memoir Problem," *Reviews in American History* 34, no. 1 (March 2006): 111.

20. Arthur W. Frank, *The Wounded Storyteller: Body, Illness, and Ethics* (Chicago: University of Chicago Press, 1995), p. 2; Hirsch quoted in Alec Wilkinson, "Finding the Words," *New Yorker,* August 4, 2014; Doris Lund, *Eric* (New York: HarperCollins, 1974), p. 6; Yagoda, *Memoir;* Anne Sexton, "The Truth the Dead Know," in *The Complete Poems* (Boston: Houghton Mifflin, 1981); Richard Lischer, *Stations of the Heart: Parting with a Son* (New York: Alfred A. Knopf, 2013), p. 51.

21. For more discussion of personal narratives as counternarratives, see Mary Jo Maynes, Jennifer L. Pierce, and Barbara Laslett, *Telling Stories: The Use of Personal Narratives in the Social Sciences and History* (Ithaca, NY: Cornell University Press, 2008), pp. 8–11, 63–69.

22. David J. Morris, *The Evil Hours: A Biography of Post-Traumatic Stress Disorder* (New York: Mariner Books, 2015), p. 66; Anemona Hartocollis, "At the End, Offering Not a Cure but Comfort," *New York Times,* August 20, 2009; Stephen S. Rosenfeld, *The Time of Their Dying* (New York: Norton, 1977), p. 177; Emily Rapp, *The Still Point of the Turning World* (New York: Penguin Press, 2013), p. 12.

23. Quoted in Elisabeth Young-Bruehl, *Anna Freud: A Biography* (New York: Summit Books, 1988), p. 377.

Chapter 1. "The Human Touch"

1. Gordon Livingston, *Only Spring: On Mourning the Death of My Son* (New York: Marlowe, 1995), p. 3.

2. Sarah Elizabeth Harrington and Thomas J. Smith, "The Role of Chemotherapy at the End of Life: 'When Is Enough, Enough?,'" *Journal of the American Medical Association* 299, no. 22 (June 11, 2008): 2667–78; Haiden A. Husskamp, Nancy L. Keating, Jennifer L. Malin, Alan M. Zaslavsky, Jane C. Weeks, Craig C. Earle, Joan M. Teno, et al., "Discussions with Physicians about Hospice among Patients with Metastatic Lung Cancer," *Archives of Internal Medicine* 169, no. 10 (May 25, 2009): 954–62; Jane C. Weeks, Paul J. Catalano, Angel Cronin, Matthew D. Finkelman, Jennifer W. Mack, Nancy L. Keating, and Deborah Schrag, "Patients' Expectations about Effects of Chemotherapy for Advanced Cancer," *New England Journal of Medicine* 367, no. 17 (October 15, 2012): 1616–25; Sissela Bok, *Secrets: On the Ethics of Concealment and Revelation* (New York: Random House, 1983).

3. American Medical Association, *Medical Ethics and Etiquette: The Code of Ethics Adopted by the American Medical Association,* with commentaries by Austin Flint (New York: Appleton, 1895), p. 21.

4. Michael Bliss, *The Making of Modern Medicine: Turning Points in the Treatment of Disease* (Chicago: University of Chicago Press, 2011), p. 35; Robert A. Aronowitz, *Unnatural History: Breast Cancer and American Society* (New York: Cambridge University Press, 2007); Keith Wailoo, *How Cancer Crossed the Color Line* (New York: Oxford University Press, 2011).

5. Louis Lasagna, "Editorial: The Doctor and the Dying Patient," *Journal of Chronic Diseases* 22 (1969): 66; Leland Christenson, "The Physician's Role in Terminal Illness and Death" (editorial), *Minnesota Medicine* 46 (September 1963): 881–82; William Kitay, "Let's Retain the Dignity of Dying," *Today's Health,* May 1966, 62–69; Samuel Standard and Helmuth Nathan, eds., *Should the Patient Know the Truth?* (New York: Springer, 1955); Mary Ann Krisman-Scott, "An Historical Analysis of Disclosure of Terminal Status," *Image* 32, no. 1 (2000): 47–52; Donald Oken, "What to Tell Cancer Patients: A Study of Medical Attitudes," *Journal of the American Medical Association* 175, no. 13 (April 1, 1961): 86–94.

6. Barney G. Glaser and Anselm L. Strauss, *Awareness of Dying* (New Brunswick, NJ: Aldine Transaction, 1965).

7. Elisabeth Kübler-Ross, *On Death and Dying* (New York: Simon and Schuster, 1969); see Emily K. Abel, "The Hospice Movement: Institutionalizing Innovation," *International Journal of Health Services* 16, no. 1 (1986): 71–85; David J. Rothman, *Strangers at the Bedside: A History of How Law and Bioethics Transformed Medical Decision Making* (New York: Basic Books, 1991).

8. Gerda Lerner, *A Death of One's Own* (New York: Simon and Schuster, 1978), pp. 57–58.

9. Joan Gould, *Spirals* (New York: Random House, 1988), p. 20.

10. Dietrich Niethammer, *Speaking Honestly with Sick and Dying Children and Adolescents: Unlocking the Silence* (Baltimore: Johns Hopkins University Press, 2012); Myra Bluebond-Langner, *The Private Worlds of Dying Children* (Princeton, NJ: Princeton University Press, 1978).

11. Terry Pringle, *This Is the Child* (Dallas: Southern Methodist University Press, 1981), p. 28.

12. Dennis H. Novack, Robin Plumer, Raymond L. Smith, Herbert Ochitill, Gary R. Morrow, and John M. Bennett, "Changes in Physicians' Attitudes toward Telling the Cancer Patient," *Journal of the American Medical Association* 241, no. 9 (March 2, 1979): 897–900; Sydney A. Halpern, "Medical Authority and the Culture of Rights," *Journal of Health Politics, Policy, and Law* 29, nos. 4–5 (August–October 2004): 835–52; Anne Harrington, *The Cure Within: A History of Mind-Body Medicine* (New York: W. W. Norton, 2008); Krisman-Scott, "Historical Analysis," 47–52; Rothman, *Strangers at the Bedside;* Carl E. Schneider, *The Practice of Autonomy: Patients, Doctors, and Medical Decisions* (New York: Oxford University Press, 1998); Robert Zussman, "Sociological Perspectives on Medical Ethics and Decision-Making," *Annual Review of Sociology* 23 (1997): 171–89.

13. Nicholas A. Christakis, *Death Foretold: Prophecy and Prognosis in Medical Care* (Chicago: University of Chicago Press, 1999); Elizabeth B. Lamont and Nicholas A. Christakis, "Prognostic Disclosure to Patients with Cancer near the End of Life," *Annals of Internal Medicine* 134, no. 12 (June 19, 2001): 1096–1105; Carol K. Oyster, "Whose Death Is It, Anyway," in *Final Acts: Death, Dying, and the Choices We Make,* ed. Nan Bauer-Maglin and Donna Perry (New Brunswick, NJ: Rutgers University Press, 2010), p. 92; Mimi Schwartz, "Elegy for an Optimist," in ibid., pp. 123–25.

14. Stan Mack, *Janet and Me: An Illustrated Story of Love and Loss* (New York: Simon and Schuster, 2004), p. 81; Laurie Foos, "On Bearing Witness," in *At the End of Life: True*

Stories about How We Die, ed. Lee Gutkind (Pittsburgh: Creative Nonfiction Books, 2011), p. 9.

15. Pringle, *This Is the Child,* p. 68; Mary Winfrey Trautmann, *The Absence of the Dead Is Their Way of Appearing* (Pittsburgh: Cleis Press, 1984), p. 10.

16. Will Schwalbe, *The End of Your Life Book Club* (New York: Knopf, 2012), p. 178; Mack, *Janet and Me,* p. 19.

17. Philip Roth, *Patrimony* (New York: Random House, 1991), p. 66.

18. Elaine Ipswitch, *Scott Was Here* (New York: Dell, 1978), pp. 41–42; see Renée Fox, *Experiment Perilous: Physicians and Patients Facing the Unknown* (Glencoe, IL: Free Press, 1959).

19. Stanford B. Friedman, Myron Karon, and Gary Goldsmith, *Childhood Leukemia: A Pamphlet for Parents* (Washington, DC: US Department of Health, Education, and Welfare, Public Health Service, 1964); Stanford B. Friedman, "Care of the Family of the Child with Cancer," *Pediatrics* 40, no. 3, suppl. (1967): 501.

20. Trautmann, *Absence of the Dead,* p. 10; Pringle, *This Is the Child,* p. 27; Kathy Davis, *The Making of "Our Bodies, Ourselves": How Feminism Travels across Borders* (Durham, NC: Duke University Press, 2007); Sandra Morgen, *Into Our Own Hands: The Women's Health Movement in the United States* (New Brunswick, NJ: Rutgers University Press, 2002); Jeffrey T. Huber and Mary L. Gillaspy, "Knowledge/Power Transforming the Social Landscape: The Case of the Consumer Health Information Movement," *Library Quarterly* 84, no. 4 (2011): 405–30; D. J. Sager, "Answering the Call for Health Information," *American Libraries* 9 (September 1978): 480–82.

21. Lynn S. Baker, *You and Leukemia: A Day at a Time* (Philadelphia: W. B. Saunders, 1978); Judith M. Chessels, "You and Leukemia—A Day at a Time," *Journal of Clinical Pathology* 32, no. 7 (July 1979): 743; Pringle, *This Is the Child,* p. 50.

22. Susannah Fox and Deborah Fallows, "Internet Health Resources," Pew Research Internet Project, July 16, 2003, www.pewinternet.org/2003/07/16/internjet-health -resources.

23. Charles C. Rosenberg, *The Care of Strangers: The Rise of America's Hospital System* (New York: Basic Books, 1987); Condict W. Cutler Jr., "Forty Years Ago," in *The Roosevelt Hospital, 1871–1957* (New York: Roosevelt Hospital, 1957), p. 170.

24. Terry Tempest Williams, *Refuge: An Unnatural History of Family and Place* (New York: Vintage, 1991), pp. 27, 205.

25. Pringle, *This Is the Child,* pp. 14–15; Mack, *Janet and Me,* p. 15.

26. Rose Levit, *Ellen: A Short Life Long Remembered* (New York: Bantam Books, 1974), pp. 80–81.

27. Richard Lischer, *Stations of the Heart: Parting with a Son* (New York: Alfred A. Knopf, 2013), pp. 45–46.

28. Mack, *Janet and Me.*

29. Alan Shapiro, *Vigil* (Chicago: University of Chicago Press, 1996), p. 26.

30. Ibid., pp. 54–56.

31. Livingston, *Only Spring,* pp 89, 97. On physicians who abandon dying patients, see Anthony L. Back, Jessica P. Young, Ellen McCown, Ruth A. Engelberg, Elizabeth K. Vig, Lynn F. Reinke, Marjorie D. Wenrigh, Barbara B. McGrath, and J. Randall Curtis, "Abandonment at the End of Life from Patient, Caregiver, Nurse, and

Physician Perspectives: Loss of Continuity and Lack of Closure," *Archives of Internal Medicine* 169, no. 5 (2009): 474–79; Pauline W. Chen, "When Patients Feel Abandoned by Doctors," *New York Times,* March 12, 2009.

32. Marcia Friedman, *The Story of Josh* (New York: Ballantine Books, 1974), pp. 264–65.

33. Frank Deford, *Alex: The Life of a Child* (Nashville: Rutledge Hill Press, 1983), p. 157.

34. Hillary Johnson, *My Mother Dying* (New York: St. Martin's Press, 1999).

35. Jacquie Gordon, *Give Me One Wish* (New York: W. W. Norton, 1988), p. 29.

36. Deford, *Alex,* p. 160; Johnson, *My Mother Dying,* p. 241.

37. Lamont and Christakis, "Prognostic Disclosure"; Pringle, *This Is the Child,* p. 184; see Beecher Grogan, "Simple Gifts," in *At the End of Life: True Stories about How We Die,* ed. Lee Gutkind (Pittsburgh: Creative Nonfiction Books, 2011), p. 76.

Chapter 2. "Hope Became a Companion in Our Home"

1. David Rieff, *Swimming in a Sea of Death: A Son's Memoir* (New York: Simon and Schuster, 2008), p. 61.

2. Ilana Löwy, *Between Bench and Bedside: Science, Healing, and Interleukin-2 in a Cancer Ward* (Cambridge, MA: Harvard University Press, 1996), p. 28; see Dan W. Brock, "The Allure of Questionable-Benefit Treatment," in *Malignant: Medical Ethicists Confront Cancer,* ed. Rebecca Dresser (New York: Oxford University Press, 2012), pp. 103–7; Andrea C. Enzinger, Bachui Zhand, Jane C. Weeks, and Holly G. Prigerson, "Clinical Trial Participation as Part of End-of-Life Cancer Care: Associations with Medical Care and Quality of Life near Death," *Journal of Pain and Symptom Management* 47, no. 6 (June 2014): 1078–90.

3. "We Could Cure Cancer Now!," *Woman's Home Companion,* November 1946, pp. 35, 176; Jordan Goodman, Anthony McElligott, and Lara Marks, "Making Human Bodies Useful: Historicizing Medical Experiments in the Twentieth Century," in *Useful Bodies: Humans in the Service of Medical Science in the Twentieth Century,* ed. Goodman, McElligott, and Marks (Baltimore: Johns Hopkins University Press, 2003), p. 13.

4. Harry M. Marks, *The Progress of Experiment: Science and Therapeutic Reform in the United States, 1900–1990* (New York: Cambridge University Press, 1997); Marcia Meldrum, "A Brief History of the Randomized Controlled Trial: From Oranges and Lemons to the Gold Standard," *Hematology and Oncology Clinics of North America* (August 14, 2000): 745–60; Paul S. Appelbaum and Charles W. Lidz, "The Therapeutic Misconception," in *The Oxford Textbook of Clinical Research Ethics,* ed. Ezekiel J. Emanuel, Christine Grady, Robert A. Crouch, Reidar K. Lie, Franklin G. Miller, and David Wendler (New York: Oxford University Press, 2008), pp. 633–44.

5. Marks, *Progress of Experiment,* p. 13; see Dresser, *Malignant;* Sydney A. Halpern, "Medical Authority and the Culture of Rights," *Journal of Health Politics, Policy, and Law* 29, nos. 4–5 (August–October 2004): 835–52.

6. See Susan L. Smith, "Mustard Gas and American Race-Based Human Experimentation in World War II," *Journal of Law, Medicine, and Ethics* 36, no. 3 (Fall 2008): 517–21; "Mayor Dedicates City Cancer Unit," *New York Times,* August 24, 1950; see Barron H. Lerner, *The Breast Cancer Wars: Fear, Hope, and the Pursuit of a Cure in Twentieth-Century America* (New York: Oxford University Press, 2001), p. 137; James T. Patterson, *The Dread*

Disease: Cancer and Modern American Culture (Cambridge, MA: Harvard University Press, 1987), pp. 195–98; Rhoads quoted in "Doctor Foresees Cancer Penicillin," *New York Times,* October 3, 1953.

7. Erika Blackstone and Jonathan D. Moreno, "A History of Informed Consent in Clinical Research," in Emanuel et al., *Oxford Textbook,* p. 597; *The Human Radiation Experiments: Final Report of the President's Advisory Committee* (New York: Oxford University Press); David J. Rothman, *Strangers at the Bedside: A History of How Law and Bioethics Transformed Medical Decision Making* (New Brunswick, NJ: Aldine Transaction, 2011; first published 1991), p. 62.

8. Julius B. Richmond and Harry A. Waisman, "Psychological Aspects of Management of Children with Malignant Diseases," *American Journal of Diseases of Children* 89 (1955): 42–47; Rudolf Toch, "Management of the Child with a Fatal Disease," *Clinical Pediatrics* 3, no. 7 (1964): 418–27.

9. John Gunther, *Death Be Not Proud* (New York: Harper and Row, 1949), p. 57. For an excellent analysis of this book, see Gretchen Krueger, *Hope and Suffering: Children, Cancer, and the Paradox of Experimental Medicine* (Baltimore: Johns Hopkins University Press, 2008), pp. 53–81; see also Janet Golden and Emily K. Abel, "'Modern Medical Science and the Divine Providence of God': Rethinking the Place of Religion in Postwar U.S. Medical History," *Journal of the History of Medicine and Allied Sciences* 69, no. 4 (2014): 580–603.

10. Gunther, *Death Be Not Proud,* pp. 30, 57–59.

11. Henry K. Beecher, "Ethics and Clinical Research," *New England Journal of Medicine* 274 (1966): 1354–60; *Human Radiation Experiments.*

12. Jade Walker, "Doris Lund," in "The Blog of Death," *www.blogofdeath.com/2003/06/29* (accessed December 13, 2014); Doris Lund, *Eric* (New York: Perennial, 1978), p. 46.

13. Lund, *Eric,* pp. 47, 51.

14. Ibid., pp. 78–79.

15. C. P. Rhoads to D. C. Morris Jacobs, June 25, 1957, folder "Memorial Hospital-SKI," box 116, Mary Lasker Papers, Rare Book and Manuscript Library, Columbia University, New York; *Human Radiation Experiments,* p. 83; Morris A. Jacobs to Abraham D. Beame, January 6, 1958, folder "Memorial Hospital," box 116, Mary Lasker Papers.

16. Peter De Vries, *The Blood of the Lamb* (Chicago: University of Chicago Press, 2005; first published 1961); see Krueger, *Hope and Suffering,* pp. 102–4; Jeremy Pearce, "Dr. Joseph H. Burchenal, 93, Who Devised Cancer-Drug Therapy, Dies," *New York Times,* March 16, 2006; "Joseph H. Burchenal: In Memoriam (1912–2006)," *Cancer Research* 66, no. 24 (December 15, 2006): 12037–38; Lund, *Eric,* pp. 127–28; Renée Fox, *Experiment Perilous: Physicians and Patients Facing the Unknown* (New Brunswick, NJ: Transaction, 1998; first published 1959), p. 139.

17. Lund, *Eric,* p. 117.

18. Ibid., p. 203; Toch, "Management of the Child," 423.

19. Lund, *Eric,* p. 205.

20. Ibid., p. 317.

21. Ibid., p. 335.

22. Susan M. Reverby, ed., *Tuskegee's Truths: Rethinking the Tuskegee Syphilis Study* (Chapel Hill: University of North Carolina Press, 2000).

23. See, e.g., Ilene Albala, Margaret Doyle, and Paul S. Appelbaum, "The Evolution of Consent Forms for Research: A Quarter Century of Changes, *IRB* 32, no. 3 (May–June 2010): 7–11; Nicholas A. Christakis, "Should IRBs Monitor Research More Strictly?," *IRB* 10, no. 2 (March–April 1988): 8–10; Bradford Gray and Robert A. Cooke, "The Impact of Institutional Review Boards on Research," *Hastings Center Report* 10, no. 1 (February 1980): 36–41; Carl E. Schneider, *The Practice of Autonomy: Patients, Doctors, and Medical Decisions* (New York: Oxford University Press, 1998), pp. 91–93. See Ruth R. Fader and Tom L. Beauchamp, *A History and Theory of Informed Consent* (New York: Oxford University Press, 1986); Rothman, *Strangers at the Bedside.*

24. See Appelbaum and Lidz, "Therapeutic Misconception."

25. Vanessa Northington Gamble, "Under the Shadow of Tuskegee: African Americans and Health Care," in Reverby, *Tuskegee's Truths,* pp. 431–42.

26. Rose Levit, *Ellen: A Short Life Long Remembered* (New York: Bantam Books, 1974), pp. 37, 63.

27. Ibid., pp. 38–39, 74, 105–6.

28. Marcia Friedman, *The Story of Josh* (New York: Ballantine Books, 1974), pp. 182–83, 209–10.

29. Mary Winfrey Trautmann, *The Absence of the Dead Is Their Way of Appearing* (Pittsburgh: Cleis Press, 1984), p. 9; Renée C. Fox and Judith P. Swazey, *The Courage to Fail: A Social View of Organ Transplants and Dialysis,* 3rd ed. (New Brunswick, NJ: Transaction, 2009), pp. 225–333.

30. Trautmann, *Absence of the Dead,* pp. 189, 199.

31. Elaine Ipswitch, *Scott Was Here* (New York: Dell, 1978), pp. 65, 111.

32. The doctor must have been at the Fred Hutchinson Cancer Research Center; Ipswitch, *Scott Was Here,* p. 122.

33. Gerda Lerner, *A Death of One's Own* (New York: Simon and Schuster, 1978), p. 74.

34. Ibid., p. 167.

35. Ibid., p. 173.

36. Ibid., p. 208.

37. Steven Epstein, *Impure Science: AIDS, Activism, and the Politics of Knowledge* (Berkeley: University of California Press, 1996); Rothman, *Strangers at the Bedside,* p. 252.

38. Paul Monette, *Borrowed Time: An AIDS Memoir* (New York: Avon Books, 1988), p. 1.

39. Ibid., pp. 92, 103.

40. Ibid., pp. 107, 211.

41. Elizabeth Cox, *Thanksgiving: An AIDS Journal* (New York: Harper and Row, 1990), p. 120; Carol Lynn Pearson, *Goodbye, I Love You* (Springville, UT: Cedar Fort, 2006), pp. 167, 172, 174.

42. Barbara Peabody, *The Screaming Room* (San Diego: Oak Tree, 1986), pp. 144, 149, 159; Susan M. Chambré, *Fighting for Our Lives: New York's AIDS Community and the Politics of Disease* (New Brunswick, NJ: Rutgers University Press, 2006), p. 145.

43. Peabody, *Screaming Room,* p. 167.

44. The doctor is quoted in Ronald Bayer and Gerald M. Oppenheimer, *AIDS Doctors: Voices from the Epidemic* (New York: Oxford University Press, 2000), p. 120; Cox, *Thanksgiving,* pp. 140–41, 152.

45. Fenton Johnson, *Geography of the Heart: A Memoir* (New York: Washington Square Press, 1996), p. 141; see Chambré, *Fighting for Our Lives*, p. 136; Mark Doty, *Heaven's Coast: A Memoir* (New York: Harper Collins, 1996), pp. 141, 147–48.

46. Jean M. Baker, *Family Secrets: Gay Sons—A Mother's Story* (New York: Harrington Park Press, 1998), pp. 105, 131.

47. Monette, *Borrowed Time*, pp. 107.

48. *National Cancer Institute's Therapy Program, Joint Hearing before the Subcommittee on Health and the Environment of the Committee on Energy and Commerce (House of Representatives) and the Subcommittee on Investigation and Oversight of the Committee on Science and Technology*, 97th Cong., 1st sess., October 27, 1981 (Washington, DC: US Government Printing Office, 1982), pp. 152, 154, 162.

49. Ibid., p. 137; L. H. Aiken and M. M. Marx, "Perspective on the Public Policy Debate," in *Hospice Programs and Public Policy*, ed. Paul R. Torrens (Chicago: American Hospital Association, 1985); see Rebecca Dresser, *When Science Offers Salvation: Patient Advocacy and Research Ethics* (New York: Oxford University Press, 2001).

50. Jean Craig, *Between Hello and Goodbye: A Life-Affirming Story of Courage in the Face of Tragedy* (Los Angeles: Jeremy P. Tarcher, 1991), pp. 17, 19.

51. John A Robertson, "Caregivers, Patients, and Clinicians," in Dresser, *Malignant*, p 141; Will Schwalbe, *The End of Your Life Book Club* (New York: Alfred A. Knopf, 2012), pp. 269, 274.

52. Sidney J. Winawer, *Healing Lessons* (New York: Routledge, 1999), p. 105.

53. Richard Lischer, *Stations of the Heart: Parting with a Son* (New York: Alfred A. Knopf, 2013), p. 56; Rieff, *Swimming in a Sea of Death*, p. 46.

54. Paul Appelbaum, Loren H. Roth, Charles W. Lidz, Paul Benson, and William Winslade, "False Hopes and Best Data: Consent to Research and the Therapeutic Misconception," *Hastings Center Report* 17, no. 2 (1987): 20; Rebecca Dresser, "The Ubiquity and Utility of the Therapeutic Misconception," *Social Philosophy and Policy* 19, no. 2 (July 2002): 281; Rieff, *Swimming in a Sea of Death*, p. 83; Robertson, "Caregivers," p. 140.

55. Amanda Bennett, *The Cost of Hope: The Story of a Marriage, a Family, and the Quest for Life* (New York: Random House, 2002), pp. 78, 97.

56. Meghan O'Rourke, *The Long Goodbye* (New York: Riverhead Books, 2011), pp. 52, 53.

57. Lischer, *Stations of the Heart*, pp. 47–48; Bennett, *Cost of Hope*, pp. 143–52.

58. Rieff, *Swimming in a Sea of Death*, pp. 62–63, 127.

59. Zygmunt Bauman, *Mortality, Immortality, and Other Life Strategies* (Stanford, CA: Stanford University Press, 1992), p. 152.

Chapter 3. When Medicine Fails

1. Anne Harrington, *The Cure Within: A History of Mind-Body Medicine* (New York: W. W. Norton, 2008), p. 18; Norman Cousins, *Anatomy of an Illness as Perceived by the Patient: Reflections on Healing and Regeneration* (New York: W. W. Norton, 1979); Bernie Siegel, *Love, Medicine, and Miracles* (New York: HarperCollins, 1986).

2. Harrington, *Cure Within*, p. 22; Sidney J. Winawer, *Healing Lessons* (New York: Routledge, 2008), pp. 56–57, 72.

3. Jean Craig, *Between Hello and Goodbye* (Los Angeles: Jeremy P. Tarcher, 1991), p. 280.

4. Barbara Peabody, *The Screaming Room* (San Diego: Oak Tree, 1986), pp. 99, 160.

5. Scott Scheiman, "Socioeconomic Status and Beliefs about God's Influence in Everyday Life," *Sociology of Religion* 71, no. 1 (2010): 25–51.

6. Ann Hood, *Do Not Go Gentle* (New York: Picador, 2000), pp. 7, 45.

7. Carol Lynn Pearson, *Goodbye, I Love You* (Springville, UT: CFI, 2006), p. 167; Mary Winfrey Trautmann, *Absence of the Dead Is Their Way of Appearing* (Pittsburgh: Cleis Press, 1984), p. 109.

8. Terry Tempest Williams, *Refuge: An Unnatural History of Family and Place* (New York: Vintage, 1991), pp. 34–35.

9. Le Anne Schreiber, *Midstream* (New York: Viking, 1990), p. 41.

10. Madeleine L'Engle, *Two-Part Invention* (New York: Harper One, 1988), p. 187.

11. Gordon Livingston, *Only Spring: On Mourning the Death of My Son* (New York: Marlowe, 1995), pp. 14–15, 18.

12. Ibid., pp. 8, 18, 25, 43.

13. Terry Pringle, *This Is the Child* (Dallas: Southern Methodist University Press, 1981), p. 72.

14. Richard Lischer, *Stations of the Heart: Parting with a Son* (New York: Alfred A. Knopf, 2013), pp. 102, 121, 182–83,

15. Sandra Butler and Barbara Rosenbaum, *Cancer in Two Voices* (Duluth: Spinsters Ink, 1991), pp. 189, 192. The book contains alternating passages from Butler and Rosenbaum.

16. Williams, *Refuge,* pp. 14, 83.

17. Wuthnow quoted in Andrew Cherlin, *The Marriage-Go-Round: The State of Marriage and the Family in America Today* (New York: Vintage, 2010), pp. 105–6; Sara M. Evans, "E-mails to Family and Friends: Claude and Maxilla—Declining Gently," in *Final Acts: Death, Dying, and the Choices We Make,* ed. Nan Bauer-Maglin and Donna Perry (Rutgers University Press, 2010), pp. 67, 71, 77, 86.

18. Roni Rabin, *Six Parts Love: A Family's Battle with Lou Gehrig's Disease (ALS)* (New York: Scribner's, 1985), p. 33.

19. Marcia Friedman, *The Story of Josh* (New York: Ballantine Books, 1974), p. 197; David Rieff, *Swimming in a Sea of Death: A Son's Memoir* (New York: Simon and Schuster, 2008), p. 135.

20. Bobbie Stasey, *Just Hold Me While I Cry* (Albuquerque: Elysian Hills, 1993), p. 46.

21. Schreiber, *Midstream,* p. 69.

22. Elisabeth Kübler-Ross, *Questions and Answers on Death and Dying* (New York: Simon and Schuster, 1974), p. 33.

23. Elisabeth Kübler-Ross, *On Death and Dying* (New York: Macmillan, 1969), p. 5.

24. Ibid.

25. Ibid., pp. 48, 143; Kübler-Ross, *Questions and Answers,* pp. 2, 162; Elisabeth Kübler-Ross, *The Wheel of Life: A Memoir of Living and Dying* (New York: Simon & Schuster, 1997), p. 163; Roy Branson, "Is Acceptance a Denial of Death? Another Look at Kübler-Ross," *Christian Century,* May 7, 1975, pp. 464–68; Larry R. Churchill, "The Human Experience of Dying: The Moral Primacy of Stories over Stages," *Soundings* 62 (1979): 24–37; Sherwin S. Nuland, *How We Die: Reflections on Life's Final Chapter* (New York: Vintage, 1993); Ron Rosenbaum, "Turn On, Tune In, Drop Dead," *Harper's,* July 1982, 32; Andrea Fontana and Jennifer Reid Keene, *Death and Dying in America* (Cam-

bridge, UK: Polity, 2009), pp. 154–56; Patrick O'Malley, "Getting Grief Right," *New York Times*, January 11, 2015.

26. Joan M. Teno, Pedro L. Gozalo, Julie W. Bynum, Susan C. Miller, Nancy E. Morden, Thomas Scupp, David O. Goodman, and Vincent Mor, "Change in End-of-Life Care for Medicare Beneficiaries: Site of Death, Place of Care, and Health Care Transitions in 2000, 2005, and 2009," *Journal of the American Medical Association* 309, no. 5 (February 6, 2013): 470–77; Maggie Jones, "At the End of Life, Denial Comes at a Price," *New York Times*, April 3, 2009; Jane E. Brody, "When Treating Cancer Is Not an Option," *New York Times*, November 19, 2012; Jacqueline H. Wolf and Kevin S. Wolf, "The Lake Wobegon Effect: Are All Cancer Patients above Average?," *Milbank Quarterly* 91, no. 4 (2013): 690–728; Miranda Fielding, "Doctors Are Notoriously Awful about Dealing with Death and Dying," www.kevinmd.com/blog/2012/10/doctors-notoriously-awful (accessed January 28, 2015).

27. Angie Drobnic Holan, "Sarah Palin Falsely Claims Barack Obama Runs a 'Death Panel,'" www.politifact.com/truth-o-meter/statements/2009/aug/10 (accessed November 13, 2014); Fielding, "Doctors"; Grassley quoted in Jill Lepore, "The Politics of Death," *New Yorker*, November 30, 2009; Robert Pear, "U.S. Alters Rule on Paying for End-of-Life Planning," *New York Times*, January 4, 2011; Paula Span, "End of 'Death Panels' Myth Brings New End-of-Life Challenges," *New York Times*, November 20, 2015.

28. Nancy E. Morden, Chiang-Hua Chang, Joseph O. Jacobson, Ethan M. Berke, Julie P. W. Bynum, Kimberly M. Murray, and David C. Goodman, "End-of-Life Care for Medicare Beneficiaries with Cancer is Highly Intensive Overall and Varies Widely," *Health Affairs* 31, no. 4 (April 2012): 786; Dartmouth Atlas, www.dartmoughatlas.org (accessed November 13, 2014); K. E. Steinhauser, E. C. Clipp, M. McNeilly, N. A. Christakis, L. M. McIntyre, and J. A. Tulsky, "In Search of a Good Death: Observations of Patients, Families, and Providers," *Annals of Internal Medicine* 132, no. 10 (May 16, 2000): 825–32; Institute of Medicine, *Improving Quality and Honoring Individual Preferences near the End of Life* (Washington, DC: National Academies Press, 2014); Thanh N. Huynh, Eric C. Kleerup, Joshua F. Wiley, Terrance D. Savitsky, Diana Guse, Bryan J. Garber, and Neil S. Wenger, "The Frequency and Cost of Treatment Perceived to Be Futile in Critical Care," *Journal of the American Medical Association* 1173, no. 20 (November 11, 2013): 1887–94; "Chronically Ill Patients Get More Care, Less Quality, Says Dartmouth Atlas: The Fix: Major Overhaul of Medicare," April 7, 2008, www.rejf.org/en/about-rwjf/newsroom; Anemona Hartcollis, "At the End, Offering Not a Cure, but Comfort," *New York Times*, August 20, 2009. But see Ezekiel Emanuel, "Better, If Not Cheaper, Care for the Dying," *New York Times*, January 3, 2013.

29. Stephen P. Kiernan, *Last Gifts: Rescuing the End of Life from the Medical System* (New York: St. Martin's Griffin, 2006), p. 247; Katy Butler, *Knocking on Heaven's Door: The Path to a Better Way of Death* (New York: Scribner, 2013), pp. 85, 207; Atul Gawande, *Being Mortal: Medicine and What Matters in the End* (New York: Metropolitan Books, 2014), p. 182; Abigail Zuger, "Don't Spoil the Ending: 'Being Mortal' Explores the Benefits of Setting Goals for Death," *New York Times*, October 6, 2014.

30. Katy Butler, *Knocking on Heaven's Door*, p. 213; Gawande, *Being Mortal*, pp. 156; Bill Keller, "How to Die," *New York Times*, October 7, 2012; Jonathan Rauch, "How Not to Die," *Atlantic*, May 2013.

31. Peter Steinfels, "Cardinal Bernardin Says He Has Inoperable Cancer," *New York Times,* August 31, 1996; Kenneth L. Woodward and John McCormick, "The Art of Dying Well," *Newsweek,* November 25, 1996.

32. Mitch Albom, *Tuesdays with Morrie* (New York: Broadway Books, 2008; first published 1997).

33. Randy Pausch and Jeffrey Zaslow, *The Last Lecture* (New York: Hyperion, 2008); Jeffrey Zaslow, "Professor Aimed 'Last Lecture' at His Children . . . and Inspired Millions," *Wall Street Journal,* online, wsj.com/news/articles/SB12170181317988564 (accessed January 27, 2015); Jeffrey Zaslow, "A Final Farewell," *Wall Street Journal,* May 3, 2008.

34. Pausch and Zaslow, *Last Lecture;* Zaslow, "Professor Aimed"; Zaslow, "Final Farewell."

35. Doris Lund, *Eric* (New York: HarperCollins, 1974), p. 29; Andrew H. Malcolm, *Someday* (New York: Alfred A. Knopf, 1991), pp. xiii–xiv; Schreiber, *Midstream,* p. 11.

36. Alan Shapiro, *Vigil* (Chicago: University of Chicago Press, 1997), p. 23; Joyce Guimond, "We Knew Our Child Was Dying," *American Journal of Nursing* 74, no. 2 (February 74): 249.

37. Lund, *Eric,* p. 29; Stan Mack, *Janet and Me: An Illustrated Story of Love and Loss* (New York: Simon and Schuster, 2004), p. 93.

38. Ann Hulbert, "To Accept What Cannot Be Helped," December 1, 2010, http://theamericanscholar.org/to-accept-what-cannot-be-helped; Mary Jumbelic, "Death as My Colleague," in *Final Acts: Death, Dying, and the Choices We Make,* ed. Nan Bauer-Maglin and Donna Perry (New Brunswick, NJ: Rutgers University Press, 2010), pp. 143, 146.

39. Kathryn Temple, "Unintended Consequences: Hospice, Hospitals, and the Not-So-Good Death," in *Final Acts: Death, Dying and the Choices We Make* (New Brunswick, NJ: Rutgers University Press, 2010), pp. 186–87, 190.

40. Ibid., p. 188.

41. Joseph Sacco, *On His Own Terms: A Doctor, His Father and the Myth of the "Good Death"* (Ashland, OR: Caveat Press, 2006), p. 114.

42. Schreiber, *Midstream,* pp. 223, 241.

43. Craig, *Between Hello and Goodbye,* pp. 30, 65, 129, 136, 175.

44. John A. Robertson, "Caregivers, Patients, and Clinicians," in *Malignant: Medical Ethicists Confront Cancer,* ed. Rebecca Dresser (New York: Oxford University Press, 2012), p. 148.

45. Mark Doty, *Heaven's Coast* (New York: Harper, 1995), p. 150.

46. Ibid., p. 168.

47. Andrea Sankar, *Dying at Home: A Family Guide to Caregiving* (Baltimore: Johns Hopkins University Press, 1991), p. 124; Doty, *Heaven's Coast,* pp. 168, 255–56.

48. Stephen Jay Gould, "The Median Isn't the Message," *Discover* 6 (June 1985): 40–42. Gould died twenty years later of an unrelated cancer.

Chapter 4. Caring by Kin

1. US Bureau of the Census, 1990, cited in Patrick P. Fox, "Role of the Concept of Alzheimer's Disease," in *Concepts of Alzheimer Disease: Biological, Clinical, and Cultural*

Perspectives, ed. Peter J. Whitehouse, Konrad Maurer, and Jesse F. Ballenger (Baltimore: Johns Hopkins University Press, 2003), p. 213; Nancy Folbre and Julie A. Nelson, "For Love or Money—or Both?," *Journal of Economic Perspectives* 14, no. 4 (Autumn 2000): 125; see Andrew J. Cherlin, *The Marriage-Go-Round: The State of Marriage and the Family in America Today* (New York: Random House, 2009), p. 91.

2. James J. Callahan Jr., Lawrence D. Diamond, Janet Z. Giele, and Robert Morris, "Responsibility of Families for Their Severely Disabled Elders," *Health Care Financing Review* 1, no. 3 (Winter 1980): 33; D. L. Rabin and P. Stockton, *Long Term Care for the Elderly: A Factbook* (New York: Oxford University Press, 1987); Daniel Callahan, "What Do Children Owe Their Elderly Parents?," *Hastings Center Report*, April 1985, pp. 32–37; Carroll L. Estes, James H. Swan, and Associates, *The Long Term Care Crisis: Elders Trapped in the No-Care Zone* (Newbury Park, CA: Sage, 1993), p. 114; Katherine L. Kahn, Emmett B. Keeler, Marjorie J. Sherwood, William H. Rogers, David Draper, Stanley S. Bentow, Ellen J. Reinisch, Lisa V. Rubenstein, Jacqueline Kosecoff, and Robert H. Brook, "Comparing Outcomes of Care before and after Implementation of the DRG-Based Prospective Payment System," *Journal of the American Medical Association* 264, no. 15 (October 17, 1990): 1984–88; Madonna Harrington Meyer and Michelle Kesterke Storbakken, "Shifting the Burden back to Families?," in *Care Work: Gender, Labor, and the Welfare State*, ed. Madonna Harrington Meyer (New York: Routledge, 2000), p. 220.

3. Jesse F. Ballenger, *Self, Senility and Alzheimer's Disease in Modern America: A History* (Baltimore: Johns Hopkins University Press, 2006); Patrick J. Fox, "From Senility to Alzheimer's Disease: The Rise of the Alzheimer's Disease Movement," *Milbank Quarterly* 67, no. 1 (1989): 58–102; Fox, "The Role of the Concept"; Marion Roach, *Another Name for Madness* (Boston: Houghton Mifflin, 1985), p. 104. Historians have argued that the goal of increasing federal support for medical research soon trumped that of providing more support for families. If family caregiving never was considered as important as medical research, however, it was always a major concern.

4. National Alliance for Caregiving and AARP, *Caregiving in the U.S.* (Washington, DC: National Alliance for Caregiving/AARP, 2009); Lynn Feinberg, "Assessing Family Caregiver Needs: Policy and Practice Considerations," AARP Public Policy Institute Fact Sheet 258, June 2012, www.aarp.org.ppi.

5. Institute of Medicine, *Retooling for an Aging America: Building the Health Care Workforce* (Washington, DC: National Academies Press, 2008), p. 247; Steven P. Wallace, Nadereh Pourat, Linda Delp, and Kathryn G. Kietzman, "Long-Term Services and Supports for the Elderly Population," in *Changing the U.S. Health Care System: Key Issues in Health Services Policy and Management*, ed. Gerald F. Kominski (San Francisco: Jossey-Bass, 2013), pp. 623–50; Steven K. Wisensale, "Two Steps Forward, One Step Back: The Family and Medical Leave Act as Retrenchment Policy," *Review of Policy Research* 20 (2003): 135–52; Lynn Friss Feinberg and Sandra L. Newman, "Preliminary Experiences of the States in Implementing the National Caregiver Support Program," *Journal of Aging and Social Policy* 18, nos. 3–4 (2006): 95–113.

6. The current (fifth) edition of the Mace and Rabins guide is *The 36-Hour Day: A Family Guide to Caring for People Who Have Alzheimer's Disease, Related Dementia, and Memory Loss*, 5th ed. (Baltimore: Johns Hopkins University Press, 2011).

7. Mayo Clinic, "Caregiver Stress: Tips for Taking Care of Yourself," www.mayoclinic .org/healthy-lifestyle/stress-management/in-depth; AARP, "10 Ways to Deal with Caregiver Stress," www.aarp.org/relationships/caregiving (accessed December 15, 2014). Evidence of the widespread appeal of those messages comes from Internet forums (also known as message boards), which operate as virtual support groups. One of the major sites where caregivers can communicate with others online is ALZConnected, sponsored by the Alzheimer's Association.

8. Barry Petersen, *Jan's Story* (Lake Forest, CA: Behler, 2010), p. 70.

9. Ibid., pp 79, 101, 103–4, 107, 119.

10. John Daniel, *Looking After: A Son's Memoir* (Washington, DC: Counterpoint, 1996), p. 85.

11. Sue Miller, *The Story of My Father* (New York: Random House, 2003), p. 143.

12. Aaron Alterra, *The Caregiver: A Life with Alzheimer's* (Ithaca, NY: ILR Press, 1999), p. 167; Eleanor Cooney, *Death in Slow Motion: My Mother's Descent into Alzheimer's* (New York: HarperCollins, 2003), pp. 25–26.

13. Alex Witchel, *All Gone: A Memoir of My Mother's Dementia with Refreshments* (New York: Riverhead Books, 2012), p. 204; Judith Levine, *Do You Remember Me? A Father, a Daughter, and a Search for the Self* (New York: Free Press, 2004), pp. 110, 155, 187.

14. Marion Deutsche Cohen, *Dirty Details: The Days and Nights of a Well Spouse* (Philadelphia: Temple University Press, 1996), pp. 30, 32, 36.

15. "HIV Surveillance—United States, 1981–2008," *Morbidity and Mortality Weekly Report*, www.cdc.gov/mmwr/preview/mmwrhtmo/ (accessed December 12, 2013).

16. "Current Trends Update: Acquired Immunodeficiency Syndrome (AIDS)—United States," *Morbidity and Mortality Weekly Report*, June 7, 1991, pp. 358–63, 369.

17. G. Thomas Couser, *Recovering Bodies: Illness, Disability, and Life Writing* (Madison: University of Wisconsin Press, 1997), pp. 170–71. Accounts that provide insight into the experiences of caregiving for members of the second group include Kate Scannell, *Death of the Good Doctor: Lesson from the Heart of the AIDS Epidemic* (San Francisco: Cleis Press, 1999), p. 170; N. G. Schiller, "The Invisible Woman: Caregiving and the Construction of AIDS Health Services," *Culture, Medicine, and Psychiatry* 17, no. 4 (December 1993): 487–512; Peter Selwyn, *Surviving the Fall: The Personal Journey of an AIDS Doctor* (New Haven, CT: Yale University Press, 2000); Abraham Verghese, *My Own Country: A Doctor's Story* (New York: Vintage, 1995); Abigail Zuger, *Strong Shadows: Scenes from an Inner City AIDS Clinic* (New York: W. H. Freeman, 1995).

18. Susan Folkman, Margaret A. Chesney, Molly Cooke, Alicia Boccerllari, and Linda Collette, "Caregiver Burden in HIV-Positive and HIV-Negative Partners of Men with AIDS," *Journal of Consulting and Clinical Psychology* 62, no. 4 (1994): 746–56; Fenton Johnson, *Geography of the Heart: A Memoir* (New York: Washington Square Press, 1996), p. 165; Bernard Cooper, *Truth Serum* (New York: Houghton Mifflin, 1988), pp. 180, 214–25.

19. Paul Monette, *Borrowed Time: An AIDS Memoir* (New York: Avon Books, 1988), p. 28; Johnson, *Geography of the Heart*, pp. 165–66.

20. See Cherlin, *Marriage-Go-Round*, pp. 116–17; Beverly Barbo, *The Walking Wounded: A Mother's True Story of Her Son's Homosexuality and His Eventual AIDS-Related Death* (Lindsborg, KS: Carlson's, 1987), p. 155.

21. Mark Doty, *Heaven's Coast: A Memoir* (New York: Harper Collins, 1996), pp. 139–40.

22. Cooper, *Truth Serum,* pp. 196–97.

23. Doty, *Heaven's Coast,* p. 156; Cooper, *Truth Serum,* pp. 219–20; Monette, *Borrowed Time,* p. 178.

24. Amy Hoffman, *Hospital Time* (Durham, NC: Duke University Press, 1997).

25. Urvashi Vaid, foreword to Hoffman, *Hospital Time,* p. ix; Hoffman quoted on p. xi; Monette, *Borrowed Time,* p. 205.

26. D. Johnston, R. Stall, and K. Smith, "Reliance by Gay Men and Intravenous Drug Users on Friends and Family for AIDS-Related Care," *AIDS Care* 7, no. 3 (June 1995): 307–20; Joseph A. Catania, Heather A Turner, Kyung-Hee-Choi, and Thomas J. Coates, "Coping with Death Anxiety: Help-Seeking and Social Support among Gay Men with Various HIV Diagnoses," *AIDS* 6, no. 9 (1992): 1003; Robert Frost, "The Death of the Hired Man," lines 118–19.

27. Carol Lynn Pearson, *Goodbye, I Love You* (Springville, UT: Cedar Fort, 2006); Marion Winik, *First Comes Love* (New York: Vintage, 1996).

28. Elizabeth Cox, *Thanksgiving: An AIDS Journal* (New York: Harper and Row, 1990), pp. 61–63.

29. Winik, *First Comes Love,* p. 98. Cox, *Thanksgiving,* p. 110.

30. Monette, *Borrowed Time,* pp. 51, 318; Johnson, *Geography of the Heart,* p. 151; Hoffman, *Hospital Time,* p. 151.

31. Jean M. Baker, *Family Secrets: Gay Sons—A Mother's Story* (New York: Harrington Park Press, 1998), pp. 43, 181; "Dr. Jean M. Baker, Obituary," *Arizona Daily Star,* August 17, 2013; Barbo, *Walking Wounded,* p. 1; Ardath H. Rodale, *Climbing toward the Light* (Emmaus, PA: Good Spirit Press, 1989), p. 180. For excellent discussions of this issue, see Couser, *Recovering Bodies,* pp. 81–176; Heather Murray, *Not in This Family* (Philadelphia: University of Pennsylvania Press, 2010).

32. Susan L. Ettner and Joel Weissman, "Utilization of Formal and Informal Home Care by AIDS Patients in Boston: A Comparison of Intravenous Drug Users and Homosexual Males," *Medical Care* 32, no. 5 (May 1994): 462; Alysia Abbott, *Fairyland: A Memoir of My Father* (New York: W. W. Norton, 2013), p. 280.

33. Marco Roth, *The Scientist: A Family Romance* (New York: Farrar, Straus and Giroux, 2012), p. 29; Monette, *Borrowed Time,* pp. 50, 78–79.

34. Cox, *Thanksgiving,* pp. 50, 195.

35. Baker, *Family Secrets,* p. 10; Monette, *Borrowed Time,* p. 219; Cox, *Thanksgiving,* p. 156.

36. Susan Bergman, *Anonymity: The Secret Life of an American Family* (New York: Time Warner, 1995); Bobbie Stasey, *Just Hold Me While I Cry* (Albuquerque: Elysian Hills, 1993), p. 60; Cox, *Thanksgiving,* p. 78. On the lingering fear of contamination, see Wendy K. Mariner, "AIDS Phobia, Public Health Warnings, and Lawsuits: Deterring Harm or Rewarding Ignorance?," *Health Law and Ethics* 85, no. 11 (November 1985): 1562–68.

37. Janet J. Kelly, Susan Y. Chu, James W. Buehler, and the AIDS Morality Project Group, "AIDS Deaths Shift from Hospital to Home," *American Journal of Public Health* 83, no. 10 (October 1983): 1433–37; Cox, *Thanksgiving,* p. 206; Roth, *Scientist,* p. 13.

38. Stasey, *Just Hold Me,* p. 145.

39. Barbara Peabody, *The Screaming Room* (San Diego: Oak Tree, 1986), pp. 60, 116.

40. C. Kreipke, M. Luborsky, and A. Sankar, "Concepts of the Good in HIV Caregiving," paper presented at the Society for Medical Anthropology Annual Meeting, San Francisco, March 2000; Andrea Sankar, "Living with Dying: A Construct for Research and Practice," paper presented at the American Gerontological Association Annual Scientific Meeting, San Francisco, 1999; Emily K. Abel, *Who Cares for the Elderly? Public Policy and the Experiences of Adult Daughters* (Philadelphia: Temple University Press, 1991).

41. Ruth Bartlett and Deborah O'Connor, "From Personhood to Citizenship: Broadening the Lens for Dementia Practice and Research," *Journal of Aging Studies* 21 (2007): 107–18; Annemarie Mol, Ingunn Moser, and Jeannette Pols, eds., *Care in Practice: On Tinkering in Clinics, Homes, and Farms* (New Brunswick, NJ: Transaction, 2010); Tom Kitwood, *Dementia Reconsidered: The Person Comes First* (New York: Open University Press, 1997); Athena McLean, *The Person in Dementia: A Study of Nursing Home Care in the US* (Peterborough, ON: Broadview Press, 2007); Steven R. Sabat, "Voices of Alzheimer's Disease Sufferers: A Call for Treatment Based on Personhood," *Journal of Clinical Ethics* 9, no. 1 (Spring 1998): 35–48; Steven R. Sabat and Rom Harré, "The Construction and Deconstruction of Self in Alzheimer's Disease," *Ageing and Society* 12 (1992): 443–61; Jeff A. Small, Kathey Geldart, Gloria Gutman, and Mary Ann Clarke Scott, "The Discourse of Self in Dementia," *Ageing and Society* 18 (1998): 291–316; John Thorndike, *The Last of His Mind* (Athens, OH: Swallow Press, 2009), p. 161.

42. Reeve Lindbergh, *No More Words* (New York: Simon and Schuster, 2001), p. 120; Floyd Skloot, *In the Shadow of Memory* (Lincoln: University of Nebraska Press, 2003), p. 194; Janelle S. Taylor, "On Recognition, Caring, and Dementia," *Medical Anthropology Quarterly* 22, no. 4 (2008): 327.

43. See Rachel Herz, *That's Disgusting: Unraveling the Mysteries of Repulsion* (New York: W. W. Norton 2012); William Ian Miller, *The Anatomy of Disgust* (Cambridge, MA: Harvard University Press, 1997); Martha C. Nussbaum, *Hiding from Humanity: Disgust, Shame, and the Law* (Princeton, NJ: Princeton University Press, 2004); Paul Rozin and April E. Fallon, "A Perspective on Disgust," *Psychological Review* 94, no. 1 (1987): 23–41; Paul Rozin, Jonathan Haidt, Clark McCauley, Lance Dunlop, and Michelle Ashmore, "Individual Differences in Disgust Sensitivity: Comparisons and Evaluations of Paper-and-Pencil versus Behavioral Measures," *Journal of Research in Personality* 33 (1999): 330–51. For a different interpretation, see Valerie Curtis, *Don't Look, Don't Touch, Don't Eat: The Science behind Revulsion* (Chicago: University of Chicago Press, 2013).

44. Alan Shapiro, *Vigil* (Chicago: University of Chicago Press, 1997), pp. 24–25.

45. Lauren Kessler, *Finding Life in the Land of Alzheimer's: One Daughter's Hopeful Story* (New York: Penguin Books, 2007), pp. 5, 9; Rozin and Fallon, "A Perspective on Disgust." Martha Nussbaum notes that the law of contagion means that "things that have been in contact continue ever afterwards to act on one another. . . . Well-washed clothing that has been worn by someone with an infectious disease is rejected, and many people shrink from all secondhand clothing." Nussbaum, *Hiding from Humanity*, p. 93.

46. Daniel, *Looking After*, p. 72.

47. Laura Furman, *Ordinary Paradise* (Houston: Winedale, 1998), p. 67.

48. Doty, *Heaven's Coast*, p. 223; Philip Roth, *Patrimony* (New York: Vintage Books, 1991), p. 172.

49. Miller, *Anatomy of Disgust,* pp. 194, 197; Neil Genzlinger, "The Problem with Memoirs," *New York Times,* January 28, 2011; Robert M. Adams, "The Reality Game," *New York Review of Books,* May 16, 1991.

50. Roth, *Patrimony,* p. 175; Doty, *Heaven's Coast,* p. 233.

51. Meryl Comer, *Slow Dancing with a Stranger: Lost and Found in the Age of Alzheimer's* (New York: HarperOne, 2014), pp. 165–69.

52. Doty, *Heaven's Coast,* p. 233; Baker, *Family Secrets,* p. 140.

53. Furman, *Ordinary Paradise,* p. 68; Rozin and Fallon, "A Perspective on Disgust," p. 38; Doty, *Heaven's Coast,* p. 233; Johnson, *Geography of the Heart,* p. 180.

54. Mary Gordon, *Circling My Mother* (New York: Pantheon, 2007), p. 216.

55. Madeleine L'Engle, *The Summer of the Great-Grandmother* (New York: Farrar, Straus & Giroux, 1974), p. 42.

56. Richard Lischer, *Stations of the Heart: Parting with a Son* (New York: Alfred A. Knopf, 2013), p. 113.

57. Alan Shapiro, *The Last Happy Occasion* (Chicago: University of Chicago Press, 1996), pp. 197–98, 221; Shapiro, *Vigil,* p. 51.

58. Nancy Fraser, *Unruly Practices: Power, Discourse and Gender in Contemporary Social Theory* (Minneapolis: University of Minnesota Press, 1989), p. 161.

Chapter 5. The Shadow Workforce in Hospitals and Nursing Homes

1. Ann Bookman and Mona Harrington, "Family Caregivers: A Shadow Workforce in the Geriatric Health Care System?," *Journal of Health Politics, Policy, and Law* 32, no. 6 (December 2007): 1005–41. Although Bookman and Harrington refer specifically to family members of geriatric patients, their comments are relevant to relatives of dying people of all ages.

2. Molly Haskell, *Love and Other Infectious Diseases: A Memoir* (Lincoln, NE: iUniverse.com, 1990), pp. 149–50.

3. Gerda Lerner, *A Death of One's Own* (New York: Simon and Schuster, 1978), pp. 40–41; Martha Weinman Lear, *Heartsounds* (New York: Simon and Schuster, 1980), pp. 23, 34.

4. Julie Fairman and Joan Lynaugh, *Critical Care Nursing: A History* (Philadelphia: University of Pennsylvania Press, 1998), p. 5; Jean-Louis Vincent, "Critical Care— Where Have We Been and Where Are We Going?," *Critical Care* 17, suppl. 1 (March 12, 2013): 52.

5. *Memorial Hospital for the Treatment of Cancer and Allied Diseases* (New York: Knickerbocker Press, 1913), pp. 87–88; David Rosner, *Once Charitable Enterprise* (New York: Cambridge University Press, 1982), p. 77; Emily K. Abel, *The Inevitable Hour: A History of Caring for Dying Patients in America* (Baltimore: Johns Hopkins University Press, 2013), pp. 50–51; David Sudnow, *Passing On* (Englewood Cliffs, NJ: Prentice-Hall, 1967), p. 46; Max C. Sadove, James Cross, Harry G. Higgins, and Manuel J. Segall, "The Recovery Room Expands Its Service," *Modern Hospital* 83, no. 5 (November 1954): 70; Athena M. Cleveland, "ICU Visitation Policies," *Nursing Management* 25, no. 9 (September 1994): 80A–80D; Jenny Hamner, "Visitation Policies in the ICU: A Time for Change," *Critical Care Nurse* 10, no. 1 (1990): 48–50.

6. Andrew H. Malcolm, *Someday* (New York: Alfred A. Knopf, 1991), p. 278; Lear, *Heartsounds,* p. 26.

7. Angela Frazier, Heather Frazier, and Nancy Warren, "A Discussion of Family-Centered Care within the Pediatric Intensive Care Unit," *Critical Care Nursing Quarterly* 33, no. 1 (January–March 2010): 82–86; Nancy E. Page and Nancy M. Boeing, "Visitation in the Pediatric Intensive Care Unit: Controversy and Compromise," *AACN Advanced Critical Care* 15, no. 3 (August 1994): 286–95; J. Young, "Changing Attitudes toward Families of Hospitalized Children from 1935 to 1975: A Case Study," *Journal of Advanced Nursing* 17, no. 2 (December 1992): 1422–29; Gordon Livingston, *Only Spring: On Mourning the Death of My Son* (New York: Marlowe, 1997), p. 156.

8. Judith Walzer Leavitt, *Make Room for Daddy: The Journey from Waiting Room to Birthing Room* (Chapel Hill: University of North Carolina Press, 2009); Catherine A. Chesla, "Reconciling Technologic and Family Care in Critical-Care Nursing," *Journal of Nursing Scholarship* 28, no. 3 (Fall 1996): 199–203; Betty L. Hopping, Scott F. Sickbet, and Joanne Ruth, "A Study of Factors Associated with CCU Visiting Policies," *Critical Care Nurse* 12, no. 2 (1992): 8–15; Donald M. Berwick, "Yale Medical School Graduation Address," New Haven, CT, May 24, 2010; Donald M. Berwick, "Restrictions on Family Presence in the ICU," letter to the editor, *Journal of the American Medical Association* 292, no. 27 (December 8, 2004): 2721–22; C. Damboise and S. Cardin, "Family-Centered Critical Care: How One Unit Implemented a Plan," *American Journal of Nursing* 103, no. 6 (2003): 56AA–56EE; Hank Post, "Letting the Family in during a Code," *Nursing* 19, no. 3 (March 1989): 43–46.

9. See, for example, A. J. Brown, "Effect of Family Visits on the Blood Pressure and Heart Rate of Patients in the Coronary Care Unit," *Heart and Lung* 5 (1976): 291–95; M. J. Gurley, "Determining ICU Visitation Hours," *Medsurg Nursing* 4 (1995): 40–43; J. T. Hepworth, S. F. Hendrickson, and J. Lopez, "Time Series Analysis of Physiological Response during ICU Visitation," *Western Journal of Nursing Research* 16 (1994): 704–17; T. Simpson and J. Shaver, "Cardiovascular Responses to Family Visits in Coronary Care Unit Patients," *Heart and Lung* 19 (1990): 344–51; Margaret A. Coultern, "The Needs of Family Members of Patients in Intensive Care Units," *Intensive Care Nursing* 5 (1989): 4–10; Mairead Hickey, "What Are the Needs of Families of Critically Ill Patients? A Review of the Literature since 1976," *Heart and Lung* 19, no. 4 (July 1990): 401–15; Janet Holden, Lynne Harrison, and Martin Johnson, "Families, Nurses and Intensive Care Patients: A Review of the Literature," *Journal of Critical Nursing* 11 (2002): 140–48; Ruth M. Kleinpell, "Needs of Families of Critically Ill Patients: A Literature Review," *Critical Care Nurse* 11, no. 8 (1991): 34–40; Nancy C. Molter, "Needs of Relatives of Critically Ill Patients: A Descriptive Study," *Heart and Lung* 8, no. 2 (March–April 1979): 332–39; S. Veraeghe, T. Defloor, F. Van Zuuren, M. Duijnstee, and M. Grypdonck, "The Needs and Experiences of Family Members of Adult Patients in an Intensive Care Unit: A Review of the Literature," *Journal of Clinical Nursing* 14 (2005): 501–9; American Association of Critical-Care Nurses, "Family Visitation in the Adult Intensive Care Unit," PracticeAlert, November 2011, www.aacn.org/WD/practice/docs/practicealerts/familyvisitation-adult-icu -practicealert.pdf.

10. "Don Berwick's Challenge: Eliminate Restrictions on Visiting Hours in the Intensive Care Unit," www.ihi.org/knowledge/Pages/ImprovementStories/ (accessed November 3, 2014); Donald M. Berwick and Meera Kotagal, "Restricted Visiting Hours in ICUs: Time to Change?," editorial, *Journal of the American Medical Association* 292 (2004): 736–37; quote in Berwick, "Yale Graduation Address."

11. See, for example, Stuart J. Younger, Claudia Coulton, Robert Welton, Barbara Juknialis, and David L. Jackson, "ICU Visiting Policies," *Critical Care Medicine* 12, no. 7 (1984): 607; Laura L. Stockdale and Jeffrey P. Hughes, "Critical Care Unit Visiting Policies: A Survey," *Focus on Critical Care* 15, no. 6 (1988): 45–48; Karin T. Kirchhoff and Nancy Dahl, "American Association of Critical-Care Nurses' National Survey of Facilities and Units Providing Critical Care," *American Journal of Critical Care* 15 (2006): 13–28; American Association of Critical Care Nurses, "Family Presence"; "Visiting Hours for Acutely Ill Neuro Pts." (1998), http://allnurses.com/neuro-intensive care/visiting-hours-acutely-6766 .html; "ICU Visitor's Policy/Visiting Hours" (2000), http://allnurses.com/ccu-nursing -coronary/icu-visitors-policy; "Open Visitation in Critical Care Units" (2003), http:// allnurses.com/south-carolina-nursing/open-visitation-critical; "ICU Visiting Hours" (2004), http://allnurses.com/neuro-intensive-care/icu-visiting-hours-136922.html; "Open Visiting Hours in ICU . . . Yes or No?" (2006), http://allnurses.com/micu-sicu -nursing/open-visiting-hours; "24-Hour ICU Visiting Hours?" (February 20, 2007), http://medscapenursing.blogs.com/medscape_nursing/2007/02/24hour; "Dealing with ICU Visitors" (2009), http://allnurses.com/micu-sicu-nursing/dealing-icu-visitors-policy -385843.html; "ICU-Visiting Hours . . . What Is Reasonable?" (2010), http://allnurses.com /micu-sicu-nursing/icu-visiting-hours-09670.html; "Total Disregard for Nursing Hours" (2012), http://allnurses.com/nurse-colleague-patient/; "24 Hour Visiting" (2012), http:// allnurses.com/critical-care-nursing/24-hour-visiting-745426.html.

12. Sandra M. Gilbert, *Wrongful Death: A Memoir* (New York: W. W. Norton, 1995), pp. 334–36.

13. "ICU Outcomes (Mortality and Length of Stay) Methods, Data Collection," http://healthppolicy.ucsf.edu/content/icu-outcomes (accessed November 12, 2014); Susan J. Diem, John D. Lantos, and James A Tulsky, "Cardiopulmonary Resuscitation on Television—Miracles and Misinformation," *New England Journal of Medicine* 334 (June 13, 1996): 1578–82; Myke S. van Gijn, Dionne Frijns, Esther M. M. van de Glind, Barbara C. van Munster, and Marjie E. Hamaker, "The Chance of Survival and the Functional Outcome after In-hospital Cardiopulmonary Resuscitation in Older People: A Systemic Review," *Age and Ageing* (2014): 108.

14. Stefan Timmermans, *Sudden Death and the Myth of CPR* (Philadelphia: Temple University Press, 1999), p. 28.

15. Post, "Letting the Family," p. 45; Jerome Groopman, "Being There," *New Yorker,* April 3, 2006, pp. 34–39; Constance J. Doyle, Hank Post, Richard E. Burney, John Maino, Marcie Keefe, and Kenneth J. Rhee, "Family Participation during Resuscitation: An Option," *Annals of Emergency Medicine* 16 (June 1987): 673–75.

16. "Emergency Nurses Association, Resolution Number 93-02," *Journal of Trauma* 48, no. 6 (2000): 1021; Theresa A. Meyers, "'Why Couldn't I Have Seen Him?,'" *American Journal of Nursing* 100, no. 2 (February 2000): 9.

17. Angela Genusa, "To Be—or Not to Be—in the ER," *Newsweek,* April 16, 1998; S. James, "Family Presence," videotape, *Dateline,* NBC Television, July 30, 1999; D. Shelton, "Opening the Emergency Room," *Washington Post,* February 17, 1998; Suzanne Sprague, "Families in the E. R.," *Weekend Edition Sunday,* NPR, May 10, 1998; S. Bonner, "The ER Hazard You Must Know About," *Redbook,* August 1998, pp. 114–15, 139–40; R. Davis, "Bedside in the ER: Hospitals Allowing Family Member Access," *USA Today,* March 7,

2000; Paul Jennings, "Family Presence," *World News Report*, ABC Television, June 13, 2001; "New Report Details Benefits of Family's Presence in Emergency Room," CNN, April 16, 2000; D. Tuller, "A Debate over Loved Ones in the ER," *New York Times*, May 15, 2001; Theresa A. Meyers, Dezra Eichhhorn, Cathie E. Guzzetta, Angela Clark, Jorie D. Klein, Ellen Taliaferro, and Amy Calvin, "Family Presence during Invasive Procedures and Resuscitation," *American Journal of Nursing* 100, no. 2 (February 2000): 32–43; American Heart Association, "Guidelines 2000 for Cardiopulmonary Resuscitation," part 2, "Ethical Aspects of CPR and ECC," *Circulation* 102, suppl. (2000): 112–12.

18. Stephen D. Helmer, R. Stephen Smith, Jonathan M. Dort, William M. Shapiro, and Brian S. Katan, "Family Presence during Trauma Resuscitation: A Survey of AAST and ENA Members," *Journal of Trauma* 48, no. 6 (2000): 1015.

19. Ibid.

20. Patricia Jabre, Vanessa Belpomme, Elie Azoulay, Line Jacob, Lionel Bertrand, Frederic Lapostolle, et al., "Family Presence during Cardiopulmonary Resuscitation," *New England Journal of Medicine* 368, no. 11 (March 14, 2013): 1008–18; Anahad O'Connor, "Letting Families Stay in the Trauma Ward," *New York Times*, May 1, 2012.

21. Arnold Relman, "On Breaking One's Neck," *New York Review of Books*, February 6, 2014; Manuel Martinez-Maldonado, "Letter to the Editors," *New York Review of Books*, May 8, 2014; Arnold Relman, "Letter to the Editors," *New York Review of Books*, May 8, 2014. Philip Roth may have drawn on his own experience at the time of his father's illness when he provided a fictional account of a similar incident. This time the relative rather than the patient was famous. In *Zuckerman Unbound*, Roth's alter ego, Nathan Zuckerman, visited his dying father in an ICU. The entire family crowded around the bedside. "Each was only to have stayed for five minutes, but because Nathan was Nathan, hospital rules had been suspended by the physician in charge." Philip Roth, *Zuckerman Bound* (containing *Zuckerman Unbound*) (New York: Farrar, Straus & Giroux, 1981), p. 362.

22. Younger et al., "ICU Visiting Policies," p. 607; comment to O'Connor, "Letting Families Stay," posted on New York Times, *Well*, http://well.blogs.nytimes.com/2012/05 /01 (accessed June 6, 2012); the quotation about W. E. Foote Hospital is in Deborah L. Shelton, "When the Patient's Life Is at Stake, Should the Family Be Allowed In?," *Washington Post*, February 17, 1998; Kelly Weller, "Selective Family Presence," letter to the editor, *American Journal of Nursing* 101, no. 10 (October 2001): 13.

23. Kay Redfield Jamison, *Nothing Was the Same: A Memoir* (New York: Alfred A. Knopf, 2009), p. 118.

24. Vicki Forman, *This Lovely Life: A Memoir of Premature Motherhood* (Boston: Houghton Mifflin Harcourt, 2009), p. 95.

25. Bruce V. Vladeck, *Unloving Care: The Nursing Home Tragedy* (New York: Basic Books, 1980); Theda L. Waterman, "Nursing Homes—Are They Homes? Is There Nursing?," *American Journal of Public Health* 43, no. 3 (1953): 308; Ellen Schell, "The Origins of Geriatric Nursing: The Chronically Ill Elderly in Almshouses and Nursing Homes, 1900–1950," *Nursing History Review* 1 (1993): 203–16; "Nursing Home Care in Maryland," *Public Health Reports* 77, no. 1 (January 1962): 89–90; Ollie A. Randall, "The Situation with Nursing Homes," *American Journal of Nursing* 65, no. 11 (November 1965): 92–97; Jerry Solon, "On Patients and Their Proprietary Nursing Homes," *Public Health Reports* 71, no. 7 (July 1956): 646–51.

26. Committee on Nursing Home Regulation, Institute of Medicine, *Improving the Quality of Care in Nursing Homes* (Washington, DC: National Academy Press, 1986); Nicholas G. Castle and Jamie C. Ferguson, "What Is Nursing Home Quality and How Is It Measured?," *Gerontologist* 50, no. 4 (August 2010): 426–42; Charlene Harrington, "Residential Nursing Facilities in the United States," *British Medical Journal* 323 (2001): 507–10; Institute of Medicine, *Improving the Quality of Long-term Care* (Washington, DC: National Academy Press, 2001); Kieran Walshe, "Regulating U.S. Nursing Homes: Are We Learning from Experience?," *Health Affairs* 20, no. 6 (November 2001): 128–44.

27. Research Department, American Health Care Association, "Trends in Nursing Facility Characteristics," December 2013, www.ahcancal.org/research; Kaiser Commission on Medicaid and the Uninsured, "Overview of Nursing Facility Capacity, Financing, and Ownership in the United States in 2011," Issue Paper, June 28, 2013, p. 2, http://kff .org/medicaid/fact-sheet/overview-of-nursing-facility-capacity-financing-and-owner ship-in-the-united-states-in-2011/. David C. Grabowski, "The Admission of Blacks to High-Deficiency Nursing Homes," *Medical Care* 42, no. 5 (May 2004): 456–64; Vincent Mor, Jacqueline Zinn, Joseph Angelelli, Joan M. Teno, and Susan C. Miller, "Driven to Tiers: Socioeconomic and Racial Disparities in the Quality of Nursing Home Care," *Milbank Quarterly* 82, no. 2 (2004): 227–56.

28. See Madonna Harrington Meyer and Michelle Kesterke Storbakken, "Shifting the Burden Back to Families? How Medicaid Cost-Containment Reshapes Access to Long Term Care in the United States," in *Care Work: Gender, Labor, and Welfare States,* ed. Madonna Harrington Meyer (New York: Routledge, 2002); K. B. Wilson, "Historical Evolution of Assisted Living in the United States," *Gerontologist* 47, special issue 3 (2007): 8–22; David G. Stevenson and David C. Grabowski, "Sizing Up the Market for Assisted Living," *Health Affairs* 29, no. 1 (2010): 35–43.

29. "The 2012 MetLife Market Survey of Nursing Home, Assisted Living, Adult Day Services, and Home Care Costs," Metropolitan Life Insurance Co., New York, 2003–14.

30. Joseph E. Gaugler, Kathleen Krichbaum, and Jean F. Wyman, "Predictors of Nursing Home Admission to Persons with Dementia," *Medical Care* 47, no. 2 (February 2009): 191.

31. Elinor Fuchs, *Making an Exit: A Mother-Daughter Drama with Machine Tools, Alzheimer's, and Laughter* (New York: Henry Holt, 2005), pp. 95, 186. The four writers who did not mention the possibility of nursing home admission included one whose relative died before the issue arose, one whose memoir ended before institutionalization seemed appropriate, and two who were able to make other arrangements they considered satisfactory until death occurred.

32. John Thorndike, *The Last of His Mind* (Athens, OH: Swallow Press, 2009), p. 51.

33. Linda McK. Stewart, *25 Months: A Memoir* (New York: Other Press, 2004), p. 237; John Daniel, *Looking After: A Son's Memoir* (Washington, DC: Counterpoint, 1996), p. 183.

34. Judith Levine, *Do You Remember Me? A Father, A Daughter, and a Search for the Self* (New York: Free Press, 2004), pp. 212, 215; Fuchs, *Making an Exit,* pp. 142–43.

35. Daniel, *Looking After,* p. 183; Elizabeth Cohen, *The House on Beartown Road: A Memoir of Learning and Forgetting* (New York: Random House, 2003), p. 74; T. J. Mattimore, N. S. Wenger, N. A. Desbiens, J. M. Teno, M. B. Hamel, H. Liu, R. Califf, A. F. Connors, J. Lynn, and R. K. Oye, "Surrogate and Physician Understanding of Patients'

Preferences for Living Permanently in a Nursing Home," *Journal of the American Geriatrics Society* 45 (1997): 818–24.

36. Stewart, *25 Months.*

37. Floyd Skloot, *In the Shadow of Memory* (Lincoln: University of Nebraska Press, 2003); Eleanor Cooney, *Death in Slow Motion: My Mother's Descent into Alzheimer's* (New York: HarperCollins, 2003), p. 25; Fuchs, *Making an Exit.*

38. Aaron Alterra, *The Caregiver: A Life with Alzheimer's* (Ithaca, NY: Cornell University Press, 1999), pp. 158–59.

39. Fuchs, *Making an Exit,* p. 159; Marion Roach, *Another Name for Madness* (Boston: Houghton Mifflin, 1985), p. 196.

40. Barry R. Petersen, *Jan's Story* (Lake Forest, CA: Behler, 2010), p. 131.

41. Levine, *Do You Remember Me?,* pp. 155, 182–83.

42. Rachel Hadas, *Strange Relation: A Memoir of Marriage, Dementia, and Poetry* (Philadelphia: Paul Dry Books, 2011), pp. 133–34, 138.

43. Cooney, *Death in Slow Motion,* pp. 140, 150, 156–57.

44. Ibid., p. 172.

45. Fuchs, *Making an Exit,* pp. 167–68; Cooney, *Death in Slow Motion,* pp. 156–57.

46. Roach, *Another Name,* p. 240; Sue Miller, *The Story of My Father* (New York: Random House, 2003), p. 139; Lucette Lagnado, *The Arrogant Years* (New York: HarperCollins, 2011), p. 330.

47. Joseph E. Gaugler, "Family Involvement in Residential Long-Term Care: A Synthesis and Critical Review," *Aging Mental Health* 9, no. 2 (2005): 105–18; Miller, *Story of My Father,* p. 139.

48. Nancy L. Mace and Peter V. Rabins, *The 36-Hour Day: A Family Guide to Caring for People Who Have Alzheimer's Disease, Related Dementia, and Memory Loss,* 5th ed. (Baltimore: Johns Hopkins University Press, 2011), pp. 496, 506–7. Jane Gross concurs. "Do not berate the staff, constantly complain, or micromanage," she advises. Quoted in Annie Murphy Paul, "How to Care for Your Mother," *New York Times,* May 27, 2011.

49. Miller, *Story of My Father,* pp. 135–36; Lagnado, *Arrogant Years,* p. 330; Virginia Stem Owens, *Caring for Mother: A Daughter's Long Goodbye* (Louisville: Westminster John Knox Press, 2007), p. 84.

50. Arthur W. Frank, *At the Will of the Body* (Boston: Houghton Mifflin, 1991), p. 105.

Chapter 6. The Evolution of Hospice Care

1. Joy Buck, "Rights of Passage: Reforming Care of the Dying, 1965–1986" (PhD diss., University of Virginia, 2005); Donna Diers, "Before Hospice: Florence Wald at the Yale School of Nursing," *Illness, Crisis, and Loss* 17, no. 4 (2009): 299–312.

2. Florence Wald, interview by Monica Mills, Oral History Archive, Connecticut Women's Hall of Fame, New Haven, CT, June 10, 2003; Hildegard E. Peplau, *Interpersonal Relations in Nursing* (New York: G. P. Putnam's, 1952); August B. Hollingshead and Fredrick C. Redlich, *Social Class and Mental Illness: A Community Study* (New York: John Wiley, 1958); Raymond S. Duff and August B. Hollingshead, *Sickness and Society* (New York: Harper and Row, 1968); see Buck, "Rights of Passage"; Diers, "Before Hospice," p. 307.

3. Wald interview.

4. David Clark, "Total Pain: The Work of Cicely Saunders and the Hospice Movement," *American Pain Society Bulletin* 10, no. 4 (2000): 13–15; Wald interview.

5. Barney G. Glaser and Anselm E. Strauss, *Awareness of Dying* (New Brunswick, NJ: Aldine Transaction, 1965); Barney G. Glaser and Anselm E. Strauss, *Time for Dying* (New Brunswick, NJ: Aldine Transaction, 1968); Jeanne C. Quint, *The Nurse and the Dying Patient* (New York: Macmillan, 1967); David Sudnow, *Passing On* (Englewood Cliffs, NJ: Prentice-Hall, 1967); Duff and Hollingshead, *Sickness and Society,* chapter 15.

6. Wald interview; on the concept of the "family as the unit of care" in nursing, see Ann L. Whall, "The Family as the Unit of Care in Nursing: A Historical Review," *Public Health Nursing* 3, no. 4 (1986): 240–49.

7. Hildegard E. Peplau, "Peplau's Theory of Interpersonal Relations," *Nursing Science Quarterly* 10, no. 4 (Winter 1991): 162; Florence and Henry Wald Papers, MS 1659, Manuscripts and Archives, Yale University Library (hereafter cited as Wald papers). The study also is discussed in Buck, "Rights of Passage," and Cynthia C. Adams, "Dying with Dignity in America: The Transformational Leadership of Florence Wald" (EdD diss., University of Hartford [CT], 2008).

8. Adams, "Dying with Dignity," p. 90; Research Record, 11-14-69, p. 3, folder 14, box 23; Research Conference, Thursday, February 1969, p. 2, folder 3, box 22; Methodology Issues, March 12, 1969, p. 82, folder 8, box 22, all three in Wald papers.

9. Conference, 11-13-69, pp. 7, 13, 17, folder 14, box 23, Wald papers.

10. Joan Craven and Florence S. Wald, "Hospice Care for Dying Patients," *American Journal of Nursing* 75, no. 10 (October 1975): 1816–22; Research Record, 11-12-69, folder 14, box 23, Wald papers.

11. Tape 13, March 10, 1969, p. 3, folder 4, box 22, Wald papers.

12. Research Record, 3-10-70, p. 7, folder 29, box 24; Verbatim Proceedings, 2-26-69, p. 21, folder 27, box 24, both in Wald papers.

13. Conference, 11-13-69, p. 20, folder 14, box 23, Wald papers.

14. Conference, 2-11-69, p. 2, folder 4, box 22; folders 4 and 5, box 22, both in Wald papers.

15. Conference, 11-13-69, p. 17, folder 14, box 23, Wald papers.

16. *To Honor All of Life: A National Demonstration Center to Protect the Rights of the Terminally Ill: The Case for Support of Hospice, Inc.,* pp. 2, 10–11, folder 23, box 3, Wald papers; see Adams, "Dying with Dignity," pp. 122–23, 131.

17. L. H. Aiden and M. M. Marx, "Perspective on the Public Policy Debate," in *Hospice Programs and Public Policy,* ed. P. R. Torrens (Chicago: American Hospital Association, 1985); Feather Ann Davis, "Medicare Hospice Benefit: Early Program Experiences," *Health Care Financing Review* 9, no. 4 (Summer 1988): 99; Lenora Finn Paradis and Scott B. Cummings, "The Evolution of Hospice in America: Toward Organizational Homogeneity," *Journal of Health and Social Behavior* 27, no. 4 (December 1986): 373.

18. R. W. Buckingham *The Complete Hospice Guide* (New York: Harper and Row, 1983).

19. *To Honor All Life,* pp. 5, 16.

20. Florence Wald, introduction to *In Quest of the Spiritual Component of Care for the Terminally Ill: Proceedings of a Colloquium,* Yale University School of Nursing, New Haven, quoted in Joy Buck, "I Am Willing to Take the Risk": Politics, Policy, and the Translation

of the Hospice Ideal," *Journal of Clinical Nursing* 18, no. 19 (October 2009): 2704; Randi Hutter Epstein, *Get Me Out: A History of Childbirth from the Garden of Eden to the Sperm Bank* (New York: W. W. Norton, 2010), p. 128.

21. P. Rossman, *Hospice: Creating New Models for the Terminally Ill* (New York: Fawcett Columbine, 1977), pp. 39, 107; John Case and Rosemary C. R. Taylor, eds., *Co-ops, Communes, and Collectives: Experiments in Social Change in the 1960s and 1970s* (New York: Pantheon Books, 1979). My discussion of hospices as counterinstitutions is taken, with significant modifications, from my article "The Hospice Movement: Institutionalizing Innovation," *International Journal of Health Services* 16, no. 1 (1986): 71–78, which was based partly on interviews with fifteen hospice administrators in Los Angeles, San Francisco, and New York City. Statements without note citations in subsequent paragraphs rely on that research.

22. Buckingham, *Hospice Guide,* p. 6.

23. *To Honor All Life,* pp. 1, 5.

24. C. T. Tehan, "Hospice in an Existing Home Care Agency," *Family and Community Health* 5, no. 3. (November 1982): 11–20.

25. MedPac Commission, "Chapter 11," *Hospice Services,* p. 285, www.medpac.gov /documents/MedPac (accessed November 15, 2014); Davis, "Medicare Hospice Benefit," p. 100.

26. Buck, "Rights of Passage," p. 249; *Implementation of the Medicare Hospice Benefit: Hearing before the Subcommittee on Health of the Senate Committee on Finance,* 98th Cong. 2nd sess., 1984 (Statement of Senator Robert Dole, member, Senate Committee on Finance); MedPac, "Chapter 11," p. 286; the anthropologist is Andrea Sankar, writing in her book *Dying at Home: A Family Guide for Caregiving* (Baltimore: Johns Hopkins University Press, 1991), pp. 6 (quote), 30; see Harold Braswell, "Death and Resurrection in U.S. Hospice Care: Disability and Bioethics at the End-of-Life" (PhD diss., Emory University, 2014).

27. National Hospice and Palliative Care Organization, *NHPCO's Facts and Figures: Hospice Care in America* (Alexandria, VA.: National Hospice and Palliative Care Organization, 2013), p. 4; MedPac, "Chapter 11."

28. Joan M. Teno, "It Is 'Too Late' or Is It? Bereaved Family Member Perceptions of Hospice Referral When Their Family Member Was on Hospice for Seven Days or Less," *Journal of Pain and Symptom Management* 43, no. 4 (April 2012): 732–38; Joan M. Teno, Michael Plotzko, Pedro Gozalo, and Vincent Mor, "A National Study of Live Discharges from Hospice," *Journal of Palliative Medicine* 17, no. 10 (2014): 1121–27.

29. Melissa D. Aldridge Carlson, Colleen L. Barry, Emily J. Cherlin, Ruth McCorkle, and Elizabeth H. Bradley, "Hospices' Enrollment Policies May Contribute to Underuse of Hospice Care in the United States," *Health Affairs* 31, no. 12 (2012): 2690–98; Joan M. Teno, quoted in Peter Whoriskey and Dan Keating, "Rising Rates of Hospice Discharge in U.S. Raise Questions about Quality of Care," *Washington Post,* August 6, 2014; MedPac, "Chapter 11."

30. Amanda Bennett, *The Cost of Hope* (New York: Random House, 2012), p. 216.

31. John Thorndike, *The Last of His Mind: A Year in the Shadow of Alzheimer's* (Athens, OH: Swallow Press, 2009), p. 196; Valerie Seiling Jacobs, "A Better Place," in *At the End of*

Life: True Stories about How We Die, ed. Lee Gutkind (Pittsburgh: Creative Nonfiction Books, 2011), pp. 105–6.

32. Sara M. Evans, "E-mails to Family and Friends: Claude and Maxilla—Declining Gently," in *Final Acts,* ed. Nan Bauer-Maglin and Donna Perry (New Brunswick, NJ: Rutgers University Press, 2009), p. 88; Katy Butler, *Knocking on Heaven's Door: The Path to a Better Way of Death* (New York: Scribner, 2013), pp. 215, 248.

33. Will Schwalbe, *The End of Your Life Book Club* (New York: Alfred A. Knopf, 2012), pp. 316–17; Thorndike, *Last of His Mind,* pp. 211–12.

34. Diane Rubin, *Caring: A Daughter's Story* (New York: Holt, Rinehart, and Winston, 1982), p. 197; Stan Mack, *Janet and Me: An Illustrated Story of Love and Loss* (New York: Simon and Schuster, 2004), p. 111; Laurie Foos, "On Bearing Witness," in Gutkind, *End of Life,* p. 20.

35. Kathryn Temple, "Unintended Consequences: Hospice, Hospitals, and the Not-So-Good Death," in Bauer-Maglin and Perry, *Final Acts,* p. 192; Hillary Johnson, *My Mother Dying* (New York: St. Martin's Press, 1999), p. 177.

36. Rubin, *Caring,* p. 196; Mark Doty, *Heaven's Coast: A Memoir* (New York: HarperCollins, 1996), p. 254.

37. Temple, "Unintended Consequences," pp. 192, 196, 198.

38. Jean Levitan, "The Family Tree," in Bauer-Maglin and Perry, *Final Acts,* p. 116.

39. Meryl Comer, *Slow Dancing with a Stranger: Lost and Found in the Age of Alzheimer's* (New York: HarperOne, 2014), pp. 190–91; Richard Lischer, *Stations of the Heart: Parting with a Son* (New York: Alfred A. Knopf, 2013), p. 185. Most hospices now accept people with diagnoses of dementia.

40. See Institute of Medicine, *Dying in America: Improving Quality and Honoring Individual Preferences near the End of Life* (Washington, DC: National Academies Press, 2014), pp. 1–11, 2–38.

Conclusion

1. Institute of Medicine, *Dying in America: Improving Quality and Honoring Individual Preferences Near the End of Life* (Washington, DC: National Academies Press, 2014), chapter 2, p. 45.

2. Ibid., chapter 3, pp. 117–220.

Index